Health Professions Education:

A Bridge to Quality

Committee on the Health Professions Education Summit

Board on Health Care Services

Ann C. Greiner, Elisa Knebel, *Editors*

INSTITUTE OF MEDICINE
OF THE NATIONAL ACADEMIES

THE NATIONAL ACADEMIES PRESS
Washington, D.C.
www.nap.edu

THE NATIONAL ACADEMIES PRESS   500 Fifth Street, N.W.   Washington, DC 20001

NOTICE: The project that is the subject of this report was approved by the Governing Board of the National Research Council, whose members are drawn from the councils of the National Academy of Sciences, the National Academy of Engineering, and the Institute of Medicine. The members of the committee responsible for the report were chosen for their special competences and with regard for appropriate balance.

Support for this project was provided by the Health Resources and Services Administration, the Agency for Healthcare Research and Quality, the ABIM Foundation, and the California Healthcare Foundation. The views presented in this report are those of the Institute of Medicine Committee on the Health Professions Education Summit, and are not necessarily those of the funding agencies.

International Standard Book Number 0-309-08723-6 (book)
International Standard Book Number 0-309-51678-1 (PDF)
Library of Congress Control Number: 2003106403

Additional copies of this report are available from the National Academies Press, 500 Fifth Street, N.W., Lockbox 285, Washington, DC 20055; (800) 624-6242 or (202) 334-3313 (in the Washington metropolitan area); Internet, http://www.nap.edu.

For more information about the Institute of Medicine, visit the IOM home page at: **www.iom.edu.**

The serpent has been a symbol of long life, healing, and knowledge among almost all cultures and religions since the beginning of recorded history. The serpent adopted as a logotype by the Institute of Medicine is a relief carving from ancient Greece, now held by the Staatliche Museum in Berlin.

"Knowing is not enough; we must apply.
Willing is not enough; we must do."
—Goethe

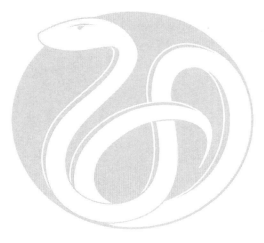

INSTITUTE OF MEDICINE
OF THE NATIONAL ACADEMIES

Shaping the Future for Health

THE NATIONAL ACADEMIES
Advisers to the Nation on Science, Engineering, and Medicine

The **National Academy of Sciences** is a private, nonprofit, self-perpetuating society of distinguished scholars engaged in scientific and engineering research, dedicated to the furtherance of science and technology and to their use for the general welfare. Upon the authority of the charter granted to it by the Congress in 1863, the Academy has a mandate that requires it to advise the federal government on scientific and technical matters. Dr. Bruce M. Alberts is president of the National Academy of Sciences.

The **National Academy of Engineering** was established in 1964, under the charter of the National Academy of Sciences, as a parallel organization of outstanding engineers. It is autonomous in its administration and in the selection of its members, sharing with the National Academy of Sciences the responsibility for advising the federal government. The National Academy of Engineering also sponsors engineering programs aimed at meeting national needs, encourages education and research, and recognizes the superior achievements of engineers. Dr. Wm. A. Wulf is president of the National Academy of Engineering.

The **Institute of Medicine** was established in 1970 by the National Academy of Sciences to secure the services of eminent members of appropriate professions in the examination of policy matters pertaining to the health of the public. The Institute acts under the responsibility given to the National Academy of Sciences by its congressional charter to be an adviser to the federal government and, upon its own initiative, to identify issues of medical care, research, and education. Dr. Harvey V. Fineberg is president of the Institute of Medicine.

The **National Research Council** was organized by the National Academy of Sciences in 1916 to associate the broad community of science and technology with the Academy's purposes of furthering knowledge and advising the federal government. Functioning in accordance with general policies determined by the Academy, the Council has become the principal operating agency of both the National Academy of Sciences and the National Academy of Engineering in providing services to the government, the public, and the scientific and engineering communities. The Council is administered jointly by both Academies and the Institute of Medicine. Dr. Bruce M. Alberts and Dr. Wm. A. Wulf are chair and vice chair, respectively, of the National Research Council.

www.national-academies.org

COMMITTEE ON THE HEALTH PROFESSIONS EDUCATION SUMMIT

Study Staff

ANN C. GREINER, Study Director, Deputy Director, Board on Health Care Services
ELISA KNEBEL, Program Officer
RACHEL COLLINS, Senior Project Assistant

Health Care Services Board

JANET M. CORRIGAN, Director
ANTHONY BURTON, Administrative Assistant
DANITZA VALDIVIA, Senior Project Assistant

Consultants

ROBERT KING, Goal QPC
RONA BRIERE, Briere Associates, Inc., Editor
ELIZABETH ARMSTRONG, Harvard Medical International and Harvard-Macy Institute
JAMES BARRON
VICKIE SHEETS, National Council of State Boards of Nursing

REVIEWERS

This report has been reviewed in draft form by individuals chosen for their diverse perspectives and technical expertise, in accordance with procedures approved by the NRC's Report Review Committee. The purpose of this independent review is to provide candid and critical comments that will assist the institution in making its published report as sound as possible and to ensure that the report meets institutional standards for objectivity, evidence, and responsiveness to the study charge. The review comments and draft manuscript remain confidential to protect the integrity of the deliberative process. We wish to thank the following individuals for their review of this report:

GERALDINE BEDNASH, American Association of Colleges of Nursing
LINDA BOLTON, Cedars Sinai Medical Center
ERIC J. CASSELL, Minisink Hills
COLLEEN CONWAY-WELCH, Vanderbilt University
DON DETMER, University of Cambridge
KEVIN GRUMBACH, San Francisco General Hospital and University of California
RALPH HALPERN, Tufts Health Care Institute
LINDA A. HEADRICK, University of Missouri-Columbia
HAROLD JONES, University of Alabama
TIMOTHY JOST, Washington and Lee University School of Law
LUCINDA MAINE, American Association of Colleges of Pharmacy
EDWARD O'NEIL, University of California
DEBRA ROTER, John Hopkins School of Public Health
GAIL WARDEN, Henry Ford Health System

Although the reviewers listed above have provided many constructive comments and suggestions, they were not asked to endorse the conclusions or recommendations, nor did they see the final draft of the report before its release. The review of this report was overseen by **Harold Fallon**, School of Medicine, University of Alabama (emerita) at Birmingham, and **Paul Griner**, University of Rochester School of Medicine and Dentistry. Appointed by the National Research Council and the Institute of Medicine, they were responsible for making certain that an independent examination of this report was carried out in accordance with institutional procedures and that all review comments were carefully considered. Responsibility for the final content of this report rests entirely with the authoring committee and the institution.

Preface

Health Professions Education: A Bridge to Quality makes the case that reform of health professions education is critical to enhancing the quality of health care in the United States. In laying the footings for this bridge, the committee that produced this report wishes to underscore that any such reform effort must encompass all health professionals, recognize each profession's contribution, and include those outside education who, to more and lesser degrees, shape what health professionals are taught.

The members of our committee represent a broad range of health-related professions and occupations, and we collectively owe a debt to the diverse group of 150 leaders who attended the Institute of Medicine's Health Professions Education Summit in June 2002 and informed our thinking. Repeatedly we heard from the working groups at the summit about the value of collaborating across the professions to understand the nature of the problems facing health professions education and the importance of designing solutions together. Many lamented the absence of existing interdisciplinary forums, and a number of the proposed strategies and actions developed by summit participants explicitly span the professions.

Although the academic environments of the various health professions generally are not interdisciplinary, practice environments are increasingly so, posing a serious disconnect. In the future, we expect more, not less, overlap and some fusion of roles. Ideally, collaboration among clinicians in practice settings draws upon each profession's strengths and therefore optimizes care for patients.

We believe the same can be true in the realm of health professions education and that it is high time to embrace a collaborative approach to educational reform. The professions and, most important, patients will be the beneficiaries.

Edward M. Hundert, M.D.
Co-Chair
March 2003

Mary Wakefield, Ph.D., R.N.
Co-Chair
March 2003

Foreword

Health Professions Education: A Bridge to Quality represents the third phase of the Institute of Medicine's quality initiative, which was launched in 1996. This initiative is central to our mission of advancing and disseminating scientific information to improve human health.

In the first phase of the IOM's quality initiative, we documented the serious and pervasive nature of the quality problem, concluding that "the burden of harm conveyed by the collective impact of all of our health care quality problems is staggering." In the second phase of our quality initiative, spanning 1999–2001, an IOM committee laid out a vision for how the system must be radically transformed in order to close the chasm that exists between what we know to be good quality care and what actually exists in practice. The committee that authored the two reports released during this phase—*To Err Is Human: Building a Safer Health System* and *Crossing the Quality Chasm: A New Health System for the 21st Century*—stressed that reform around the margins would be inadequate.

Phase three of the quality initiative is focused on implementing the vision of a future health system laid out in *Crossing the Quality Chasm*, a system characterized by an unrelenting focus on reducing the burden of illness, injury, and disability, and thereby enhancing the health status, functionality, and satisfaction of the U.S. population. The IOM is not alone in trying to make this vision a practical reality, and acknowledges the dedication and hard work of a vast array of organizations focused on redesigning care delivery, implementing innovative financing, and seeking to standardize information technology platforms, among other efforts.

Implementing such a vision cannot be done without skilled personnel. Just as the health system must be transformed in order to advance quality, so must health professions education. The initial blueprint for such a transformation can be found in the following pages. It is a guide produced by a knowledgeable and diverse IOM committee, which benefited from the wisdom of an interdisciplinary group of experts who offered their advice at an IOM Health Professions Summit held this past June. Our hope is that this guide will aid anyone dedicated to reforming health professions education.

Harvey Fineberg, M.D., PhD
President, Institute of Medicine
March 2003

Acknowledgments

The Committee on the Health Professions Education Summit wishes to acknowledge the many people whose contributions and support made this report possible.

A number of experts in federal departments, federal agencies, and other organizations were important sources of information, generously giving their time and knowledge to further the committee's aims. The project proposal was developed by Richard Diamond, formerly of the Dental and Special Projects Branch, Division of Medicine and Dentistry, and Madeline Hess, Nursing Special Initiatives and Program Systems Branch, Bureau of Health Professions, within the Health Resources and Services Administration, Department of Health and Human Services. They were aided in planning the project by Elaine Cohen, Forest Calico, and Patricia Calico, all of the Health Resources and Services Administration.

The summit was expertly facilitated by Robert King, Goal QPC, and thirteen other facilitators who work for or with Mr. King. Heidi Hess, Kaiser Family Foundation, graciously facilitated webcasts and transcripts of the summit, which are freely accessible at www.kaisernetwork.org.

The committee commissioned two papers that provided important background information and insights for this report. Vickie Sheets, National Council of State Boards of Nursing, authored a very helpful paper on accreditation and licensure. Elizabeth Armstrong, Harvard Medical International and Harvard-Macy Institute, and James Barron authored a paper on case studies of cultural reform, which served as the basis for several of the case examples highlighted in the report. Additionally, Loretta Heuer, University of North Dakota College of Nursing and Migrant Health Service, and Thomas Maddox, Gustav Leinhard Fellow in Health Sciences Policy Institute of Medicine, provided valuable input for the report's vignettes.

The committee also benefited from the work of other committees and staff of the Institute of Medicine that conducted studies referenced in this report, in particular, the committee on Quality of Health Care in America, which produced the 2001 report *Crossing the Quality Chasm: A New Health System for the 21st Century*.

Finally, the committee wishes to acknowledge the public and private organizations that provided support for the summit and follow up report, namely the Health Resources and Services Administration (HRSA), the Agency for Healthcare Research and Quality (AHRQ), the ABIM Foundation, and the California HealthCare Foundation (CHCF).

HRSA, part of the U.S. Department of Health and Human Services, directs programs that improve the nation's health by expanding access to comprehensive, quality health care for all Americans. AHRQ, also part of the U.S. Department of Health and Human Services, provides evidence-based information on health care outcomes, quality, cost, use, and access to help people make more informed decisions and improve the quality of health care services. The ABIM Foundation is a nonprofit organization whose mission is to advance medical professionalism and physician leadership in quality improvement and assessment. And, the CHCF is a nonprofit philanthropic organization whose mission is to expand access to affordable, quality health care for underserved individuals and communities, and to promote fundamental improvements in the health status of the people in California.

Contents

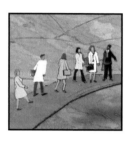 # Executive Summary

ABSTRACT

The 2001 Institute of Medicine report *Crossing the Quality Chasm: A New Health System for the 21ˢᵗ Century* recommended that an interdisciplinary summit be held to develop next steps for reform of health professions education in order to enhance patient care quality and safety. In June 2002, the IOM convened this summit, which included 150 participants across disciplines and occupations. This follow-up report focuses on integrating a core set of competencies—patient-centered care, interdisciplinary teams, evidence-based practice, quality improvement and informatics—into health professions education.

The report's recommendations include a mix of approaches related to oversight processes, the training environment, research, public reporting, and leadership. The recommendations targeting oversight organizations include integrating core competencies into accreditation, and credentialing processes across the professions. The goal is an outcome-based education system that better prepares clinicians to meet both the needs of patients and the requirements of a changing health system.

Education for the health professions is in need of a major overhaul. Clinical education simply has not kept pace with or been responsive enough to shifting patient demographics and desires, changing health system expectations, evolving practice requirements and staffing arrangements, new information, a focus on improving quality, or new technologies (Institute of Medicine, 2001):

- Health professionals are not adequately prepared—in either academic or continuing education venues—to address shifts in the nation's patient population (Cantillon and Jones, 1999; Council on Graduate Medical Education, 1999; Davis et al., 1999; Grantmakers in Health, 2001; Halpern et al., 2001; Health Resources and Services Administration, 1999; Pew Health Professions Commission, 1995). Patients in America are becoming more diverse, are aging, and are increasingly afflicted by one or more chronic illnesses, while at the same time being more likely to seek out health information (Calabretta, 2002; Frosch and Kaplan, 1999; Gerteis et al., 1993; Mansell et al., 2000; Mazur and Hickam, 1997; Wu and Green, 2000). This changing landscape requires that clinicians be skilled in responding to varying patient expectations and values; provide ongoing patient management; deliver and coordinate care across teams, settings, and time frames; and support patients' endeavors to change behavior and lifestyle—training for which is in short supply in today's clinical education settings (Calabretta, 2002).

- Once in practice, health professionals are asked to work in interdisciplinary teams, often to support those with chronic conditions, yet they are not educated together or trained in team-based skills.

- These same clinicians are confronted with a rapidly expanding evidence base—upon which health care decisions should ideally be made—but are not consistently schooled in how to search and evaluate this evidence base and apply it to practice (American Association of Medical Colleges, 1999; Detmer, 1997; Green, 2000; Shell, 2001).

- Although there is a spotlight on the serious mismatch between what we know to be good quality care and the care that is actually delivered, students and health professionals have few opportunities to avail themselves of coursework and other educational interventions that would aid them in analyzing the root causes of errors and other quality problems and in designing systemwide fixes (Baker et al., 1998; Buerhaus and Norman, 2001).

- While clinicians are trained to use an array of cutting-edge technologies related to care delivery, they often are not provided a basic foundation in informatics (Gorman et al., 2000; Hovenga, 2000). Training in this area would, for example, enable clinicians to easily access the latest literature on a baffling illness faced by one of their patients or to use computerized order entry systems that automatically flag pharmaceutical contraindications and errors.

While there are notable pockets of innovation—settings in which clinicians are being trained for a 21st-century health care system—these are by and large exceptions to the rule.

Building a Bridge to Cross the Quality Chasm

Numerous recent studies have led to the conclusion that "the burden of harm conveyed by the collective impact of all of our health care quality problems is staggering" (Chassin et al., 1998:1005). Errors lead to tens of thousands of Americans dying each year, and hundreds of thousands suffering or becoming sick as a result of nonfatal injuries. Other studies have documented pervasive overuse, misuse, and underuse of services (Chassin et al., 1998; Institute of Medicine, 2000; President's Advisory Commission on Consumer Protection and Quality in the Health Care Industry, 1998a; Schuster et al., 1998).

Crossing the Quality Chasm: A New Health System for the 21st Century (Institute of Medicine, 2001) emphasizes that safety and quality problems exist largely because of system problems, and that browbeating health professionals to just try harder is not the answer to addressing the system's flaws and future challenges. Quality problems are occurring in the hands of health professionals highly dedicated to doing a good job, but working within a system that does not adequately prepare them, or support them once they are in practice, to achieve the best for their patients.

The *Quality Chasm* report concludes that reform around the edges will not solve the quality problem, and sets forth an ambitious agenda for redesign of the broken health care system to achieve six national quality aims: safety, effectiveness, patient-centeredness, timeliness, efficiency, and equity. Implementing such an agenda has important implications for current and future health professionals. The *Quality Chasm* report provides initial guidance on what kinds of competencies clinicians would need to carry out this agenda, and emphasizes further study to better understand how the workforce should be educated for practice, how it should be deployed, and how it should be held accountable.

Health Professions Education Summit

The *Quality Chasm* report recommends that a multidisciplinary summit of leaders within the health professions be held to discuss and develop strategies for restructuring clinical education across the full continuum of education. The Committee on the Health Professions Education Summit was convened to plan and hold this summit—which was held on June 17–18, 2002—and to produce this follow-up report.

The committee organized a multidisciplinary summit involving allied health, nursing, medical, and pharmacological educators and students; health professional and industry association representatives; regulators and representatives of certifying organizations; providers; consumers; innovators in education and practice settings; and influential policy makers. Participants were asked to develop proposed strategies and actions for addressing the five competency areas recommended by the committee (described below) in health professions education: patient-centered care, interdisciplinary teams, evidence-based practice, quality improvement, and informatics.

Summit participants worked in small interdisciplinary groups using the Hoshin method (Counsell et al., 1999; Hyde and Vermillion, 1996; Platt and Laird, 1995), a structured facilitation process for gathering expert opinion and identifying, prioritizing, and implementing strategies. The ideas generated at the summit are included in this report in Appendix B. The committee conducted a literature review related to the core competencies and various recommendations that were considered. The committee also reviewed the over 200 ideas proposed by summit participants as part of its deliberations.

A New Vision for Health Professions Education

With the ideal 21st-century health care system described in the *Quality Chasm* report as a backdrop, the committee developed a new vision for clinical education in the health professions that is centered on a commitment to, first and foremost, meeting patients' needs. The committee believes that the following should serve as an overarching vision for all programs and institutions engaged in the clinical education of health professionals, and further that such organizations should develop operating principals that will allow this vision to be achieved.

All health professionals should be educated to deliver patient-centered care as members of an interdisciplinary team, emphasizing evidence-based practice, quality improvement approaches, and informatics.

The committee's vision is apparent in selected institutions—both academic and practice settings—around the country, but is not incorporated into the basic fabric of health professions education, nor is it supported by oversight processes or financing arrangements. Accordingly, the committee proposes a set of five core competencies that all clinicians should possess, regardless of their discipline, to meet the needs of the 21st-century health system. Competencies are defined here as the habitual and judicious use of communication, knowledge, technical skills, clinical reasoning, emotions, values, and reflection in daily practice (Hundert et al., 1996).

- *Provide patient-centered care*—identify, respect, and care about patients' differences, values, preferences, and expressed needs; relieve pain and suffering; coordinate continuous care; listen to, clearly inform, communicate with, and educate patients; share decision making and management; and continuously advocate disease prevention, wellness, and promotion of healthy lifestyles, including a focus on population health.

- *Work in interdisciplinary teams*—cooperate, collaborate, communicate, and integrate care in teams to ensure that care is continuous and reliable.

- *Employ evidence-based practice*—integrate best research with clinical expertise and patient values for optimum care, and participate in learning and research activities to the extent feasible.

- *Apply quality improvement*—identify errors and hazards in care; understand and implement basic safety design principles, such as standardization and simplification; continually understand and measure quality of care in terms of structure, process, and outcomes in relation to patient and community needs; and design and test interventions to change processes and systems of care, with the objective of improving quality.

- *Utilize informatics*—communicate, manage knowledge, mitigate error, and support decision making using information technology.

Many efforts have arisen in response to the need to prepare clinicians for a changing practice environment (ABIM Foundation, 2002; Accreditation Council for Graduate Medical Education, 1999; American Association of Medical Colleges, 2001; Brady et al., 2001; Center for the Advancement of Pharmaceutical Education [CAPE] Advisory Panel on

Educational Outcomes, 1998; Halpern et al., 2001; O'Neil and the Pew Health Professions Commission, 1998). To formulate the above core competencies, the committee examined the skills outlined in the *Quality Chasm* report, reviewed other efforts to define core competencies within and across the health professions, and reviewed the relevant literature.

The five competencies are meant to be core, but should not be viewed as an exhaustive list. The committee recognizes that there are many other competencies that health professionals should possess, such as a commitment to lifelong learning, but believes those listed above are the most relevant across the clinical disciplines; advance the vision in the *Quality Chasm* report; and overlap with recent, existing efforts to define competencies (Accreditation Council for Graduate Medical Education, 1999; Accreditation Council on Pharmaceutical Education, 2000). The committee also acknowledges that the core competencies will differ in application across the disciplines.

Next Steps

With some notable exceptions (O'Neil and the Pew Health Professions Commission, 1998; Pew Health Professions Commission, 1995), most current and past reform efforts have focused within a particular profession (Bellack and O'Neil, 2000; Christakis, 1995; Harmening, 1999; Jablonover et al., 2000). The committee believes the time has come for leaders across the professions to work together on the cross-cutting changes that must occur to effect reform in clinical education and related training environments, and that they should carefully consider the cultural changes necessary to support such reform efforts.

The committee believes that integrating a core set of competencies—one that is shared across the professions—into the health professions oversight spectrum would provide the most leverage in terms of reform of health professions education. A recent article synthesizing nine major reports on physician competencies, focused on the important role oversight organizations can play, concluded that "without data about medical-education quality, accreditation is the most potent lever for curricula reform in our decentralized medical education system" (Halpern et al., 2001). Many participants at the IOM summit concurred with this conclusion. The two levers for change most often cited by the 150 participants were oversight approaches and changes to financing.

The committee also recommends pursing other leverage points—such as the use of report cards that incorporate education-related measures and innovations in financial incentives—but the preponderance of its recommendations are directed at oversight organizations. This is the case in part because of the lack of education measures and the charge to this committee, which is focused on clinical education.[1] Also, health professions oversight processes, such as accreditation and certification, function at the national level, thereby affording a leverage point for systemwide change. The committee believes that such an approach will stimulate efforts on the part of educational institutions and professional associations.

The committee would like to highlight its definition of "oversight processes" and underscore that it includes the efforts of both private – and public – sector organizations:

Oversight processes include accreditation, certification, and licensure. Educational accreditation serves as a leverage point for the inclusion of particular educational content in a curriculum. Licensure assesses that a student has understood and mastered formal curricula. Certification seeks to ensure that a practitioner maintains competence in a given area over time. Organizational accreditation also may influence practitioners' ongoing competency.

The call for accrediting and certifying organizations to move toward a competency-

based approach to education is in response to growing concerns about patient safety (Institute of Medicine, 2000), the persistent and substantial variation in patient care across geographic settings that does not relate to patient characteristics (O'Connor et al., 1996; Wennberg, 1998), and the related desire on the part of public payers and consumers for increased accountability (Leach, 2002; Lenburg et al., 1999). Competency-based education focuses on making the learning outcomes for courses explicit and on evaluating how well students have mastered these outcomes or competencies (Harden, 2002). The evidence base on the efficacy of various educational approaches is slim. However, the limited evidence that does exist points to improvements, such as better performance on licensing exams, associated with the use of competency– or outcome-based educational approaches (Carraccio et al., 2002).

A competency-based approach to education could result in better quality because educators would begin to have information on outcomes, which could ultimately lead to better patient care. Defining a core set of competencies across educational oversight processes could also reduce costs as a result of better communication and coordination, with processes being streamlined and redundancies reduced. Integrating core competencies into oversight processes would likely provide the impetus for faculty development, curricular reform, and leadership activities.

Common Language and Adoption of Core Competencies

Before steps can be taken to integrate a core set of competencies into oversight processes, an interdisciplinary group that includes leaders from the professions, educational institutions, and oversight organizations will need to define common terms. A number of studies have shown that any collective movement to reform education must begin by defining a shared

---

[1] A current Institute of Medicine study addressing academic health centers is considering financing questions.

language (Halpern et al., 2001; Harden, 2002). Such an effort can help set in motion a process focused on achieving a threshold level of consensus across the disciplines around a core set of competencies.

The lack of consensus across the professions around language and terms related to the core competencies may be undermining their integration into oversight processes. For example, with respect to evidence-based practice, leaders in the field have worked to expand the definition of evidence so it includes qualitative research and to dispel the myth that such practice ignores clinical experience and expertise (Guyatt, 1992). Despite these efforts, a review of the literature suggests that misconceptions regarding the definition of evidence persist (Ingersoll, 2000; Marwick, 2000; Mazurek, 2002; Mitchell, 1999; Satya-Murti, 2000; Woolf, 2000). A review of the literature related to teaching interdisciplinary team skills reveals differing terminologies as an obstacle: faculty struggle to understand other professions' core concepts and content, which leads to conflict when they teach interdisciplinary courses (Lavin et al., 2001; Pomeroy and Philp, 1994). The committee believes that an interdisciplinary group, created under the auspices of the Department of Health and Human Services (DHHS), should be charged with developing a common language across the health disciplines and achieving consensus around a core set of competencies.

Recommendation 1: DHHS and leading foundations should support an interdisciplinary effort focused on developing a common language, with the ultimate aim of achieving consensus across the health professions on a core set of competencies that includes patient-centered care, interdisciplinary teams, evidence-based practice, quality improvement, and informatics.

Integrating competencies into oversight processes

The extent of integration of competencies into existing oversight processes varies. Any effort at further integration would be strengthened if predicated on a core a set of competencies—competencies with universal definitions shared across the professions. The committee recognizes that these competencies are by no means exhaustive, but represent an important core of what health professionals need to know to practice in a 21st-century health system.

During the last decade, competencies have begun to redefine accreditation, particularly in pharmacy and medicine. The competencies that these disciplines have defined overlap with the core competencies recommended by the committee. In 1997, the American Council on Pharmaceutical Education (ACPE) adopted accreditation standards focused on 18 professional competencies (American Council on Pharmaceutical Education, 2002). In 1999, the Accreditation Council for Graduate Medical Education (ACGME) and the organization of certifying boards, the American Board of Medical Specialties (ABMS), endorsed six general competencies as the foundation for all graduate medical education, and these competencies are currently being phased in (Accreditation Council for Graduate Medical Education, 2002). Until they are fully incorporated and evaluated, it remains to be seen what effect these competencies will have on pharmacological and medical education. In nursing, the two accrediting organizations also have defined competencies—which do not fully overlap with the core competencies defined here—but differ in whether they require demonstration of such competencies (Commission on Collegiate Nursing Education, 2002; National League for Nursing Accrediting Commission, 2002). Finally, the curricula for the selected allied health professions examined in this report vary in the extent to which they incorporate the five competencies outlined above (Collier, 2002).

The competency movement, however, does

not have as much of a foothold in licensure and certification processes. Requirements for maintaining a license vary considerably, as do requirements for those who pursue recognition of clinical excellence. Further, research has raised questions about the efficacy of continuing education courses, the most common way to demonstrate ongoing competency (Cantillon and Jones, 1999; Davis et al., 1999).

Efforts to incorporate a core set of competencies across the professions into the full oversight framework—accreditation, licensing, and certification—would need to occur on the national, state, and local levels; coordinate both public- and private-sector oversight organizations; and solicit broad input. Again, the involvement of DHHS, and specifically the Health Resources and Services Administration, would be important in getting this effort off the ground, in helping to establish a process for soliciting input from professional associations and the education community, and in identifying linkages and synergies across the various oversight groups within and across professions.

It is imperative to have such linkages among accreditation, certification, and licensure; it would mean very little, for example, if accreditation standards set requirements for educational programs, and these requirements were not then reinforced through testing on the licensing exam. All processes must be linked so they are focused on the same outcome—the ability of professionals to provide the highest quality of care.

Recommendation 2: DHHS should provide a forum and support for a series of meetings involving the spectrum of oversight organizations across and within the disciplines. Participants in these meetings would be charged with developing strategies for incorporating a core set of competencies into oversight activities, based on definitions shared across the professions. These meetings would actively solicit the input of health

professions associations and the education community.

Strategies for incorporating the competencies into oversight processes would necessarily differ across the oversight framework based on history, regulatory approach, and structure. In all cases, the oversight bodies should proceed with deliberation, with efforts made to solicit comments on draft language, and initial testing of new requirements, such as through the use of provisional standards. Processes should also be established to monitor and evaluate new requirements to ensure that they are useful and not overly burdensome.

The experiences of ACPE and ACGME provide some guidance on how accrediting bodies could incorporate competencies into their processes. Both ACPE and ACGME undertook an intensive, decade-long process of rethinking how they were preparing professionals for practice. They concluded that fundamental change was necessary, and that they needed to move away from approaches that had become increasingly precise, prescriptive, and burdensome (Byrd, 2002; Batalden et al., 2002, Leach, 2002).

What has not yet occurred is coordination across accrediting bodies of the various professions in defining a core set of competencies and related standards and measures. Such coordination would obviate the need for each accrediting body to reinvent the wheel, promote synergies, and enable better communication and working relationships, as well as more consistent integration of the core competencies across schools. This sort of coordinated effort would also help ensure that educational innovators would not be stifled by outdated accreditation requirements. Organizational accreditors—such as the Joint Commission on Accreditation of Healthcare Organizations (JCAHO) and the National Committee for Quality Assurance (NCQA)—should likewise consider more fully how clinicians maintain competency in the core set of competencies outlined above.

Recommendation 3: Building upon previous efforts, accreditation bodies should move forward expeditiously to revise their standards so that programs are required to demonstrate—through process and outcome measures—that they educate students in both academic and continuing education programs in how to deliver patient care using a core set of competencies. In so doing, these bodies should coordinate their efforts.

With the exception of patient-centered care, which is consistently included in examinations across the professions, licensing exams for health professionals vary considerably in whether they test for competency in the core areas (National Association of Boards of Pharmacy, 2002; National Council of State Boards of Nursing, 2001; United States Medical Licensing Exam, 2002). This situation also needs to be addressed and could be the focus of a subset of the oversight organizations described in recommendation 2.

In addition, geographic restrictions on licensure and separate and sometimes conflicting scope-of-practice acts need to be examined to determine whether they are a serious barrier to the full integration of the core competencies into practice, and if so, how to modify them so that all clinicians can practice to the fullest extent of their technical training and ability. Although beyond the scope of this report, the committee believes that this matter deserves further examination because licensure and scope of practice influence how clinicians are deployed, which in turn affects decisions about education. For example, licensure restrictions might hamper a rural hospital's ability to consult a specialist because she happened to be located in another state and licensed to practice only there (Phillips et al., 2002). Similarly, scope-of-practice restrictions in one state might prohibit a nurse practitioner who was part of an interdisciplinary diabetes care management team from prescribing medications, while another state might allow such activity—even though both practitioners worked for the same national health plan (Phillips et al., 2002). These restrictions make less and less sense as health care organizations and health professionals cross state lines.

Finally, the committee believes that there should be a focused effort to integrate a core set of competencies into oversight processes focused on practicing clinicians. Such an effort would require coordination among an array of public- and private-sector licensing and certification organizations, within which there is currently little uniformity in approach across the professions or within a given profession across the states. At present, many boards require only a fee for license renewal (Swankin, 2002b; Yoder-Wise, 2002), and many others view continuing education courses as evidence of competence, even though, as noted above, this has not been shown to be a reliable measure of such ability (Davis et al., 2000; O'Brien et al., 2001).

To begin with, state legislatures would need to require state licensing boards to insist that their licensees demonstrate competence, not just pay a license renewal fee, to maintain their authority to practice. To date, state legislators have not insisted upon such a requirement, in part because there is disagreement about what constitutes evidence of competency, how often it should be demonstrated, and who should judge. Licensing boards also would need to consider clinician competency at varying career stages. For example, a veteran intensive care nurse or physician subspecialist should be expected to have a higher level of competence than a new graduate in either profession.

The committee believes that all health professions boards need to require demonstration of continued competency, and that they should move toward adopting rigorous tests for this purpose. Beyond licensure examinations, there is evidence to suggest that structured direct observation using standardized patients, peer assessments, and case– and essay-based questions are reliable ways to assess competency (Epstein and Hundert, 2002; Murray et al., 2000).

Recommendation 4: All health professions boards should move toward requiring licensed health professionals to demonstrate periodically their ability to deliver patient care—as defined by the five competencies identified by the committee—through direct measures of technical competence, patient assessment, evaluation of patient outcomes, and other evidence-based assessment methods. These boards should simultaneously evaluate the different assessment methods.

There is more uniformity among certifying organizations as compared with professional boards, in that nearly all require some means of demonstrating continuing competence. The vast majority allow for two or more approaches, and many also consider competency at various career stages. Moreover, in response to the paucity of evidence that taking continuing education courses improves practice outcomes, some certifying organizations are beginning to emphasize alternative measures that are more evidence based (American Board of Medical Specialties, 2000; American Nurses Association/NursingWorld.Org, 2001; Bashook et al., 2000; Board of Pharmaceutical Specialties, 2002; Federation of State Medical Boards, 2002; Finocchio et al., 1998; National Council of State Boards of Nursing, 1997-2000; Swankin, 2002a). Although such efforts are challenging to implement and often costly, certification bodies should only recognize continuing education courses as a valid method of maintaining competence if there is an evidence-based assessment of such courses; if clinicians select courses based on an assessment of their individual skills and knowledge; and if clinicians then demonstrate, through testing or other methods, that they have learned the course content.

The committee recognizes that there is a monetary and human resource cost to moving to evidence-based assessment, whether it is related to licensure or certification. Consequently, such assessments may need to be phased in, or less

costly assessment methods identified. The committee also recognizes that increased investment in computer-based clinical records would provide the kind of rich clinical data necessary to fully realize this approach.

Recommendation 5: Certification bodies should require their certificate holders to maintain their competence throughout the course of their careers by periodically demonstrating their ability to deliver patient care that reflects the five competencies, among other requirements.

Training Environments

Education does not occur in a vacuum; indeed, much of what is learned lies outside of formal academic coursework. A "hidden curriculum" of observed behavior, interactions, and the overall norms and culture of a student's training environments are extremely powerful in shaping the values and attitudes of future health professionals. Often, this hidden curriculum contradicts what is taught in the classroom (Ferrill et al., 1999; Hafferty, 1998; Maudsley, 2001).

Consequently, the committee believes that initial support should be provided for existing exemplary practice organizations that partner with educational institutions, and are already providing the interdisciplinary education and training necessary for staff to consistently deliver care that incorporates the core competencies. Further, the committee believes that these leading organizations should be identified as training models for other organizations, and should be given the resources necessary to open their doors to students, clinicians, and faculty from other organizations, as well as support for testing alternative approaches to providing curricula that integrate the core competencies. Given that faculty shortages and lack of preparedness are a barrier to implementing some of the core competencies (Griner and Danoff, 2000; Halpern, 1996; Weed and Weed, 1999) attention should be given to faculty development as well as instruction of students.

These learning centers could test various approaches for incorporating the core competencies into education for students, clinicians, and faculty, and provide guidance to practice and educational organizations about key operational issues. Is problem-based learning the best approach to teaching these competencies? Should the teaching of these competencies be infused into other courses, or should they be stand-alone? In terms of staging, when should these competencies be taught? These learning centers should also consider how, after an initial investment, they could become self–sustaining in 3–5 years. Such a model might include provision of health care services or require outside clinicians and faculty to pay for training.

There is precedence for focusing on learning centers that span occupations. For example, in health care there are selected examples of area health education centers (AHECs) training a broad range of professionals with support from the HRSA, while in other sectors, such as the airline industry, there are more comprehensive interdisciplinary training efforts (O'Neil and the Pew Health Professions Commission, 1998). Such organizations could provide centralized locations for information technology infrastructure, which would be an efficient way of aggregating costs across many organizations.

Recommendation 6: Foundations, with support from education and practice organizations, should take the lead in developing and funding regional demonstration learning centers, representing partnerships between practice and education. These centers should leverage existing innovative organizations and be state-of-the art training settings focused on teaching and assessing the five core competencies.

There are many barriers to incorporating the five competencies into the practice environment, where medical residents and new graduates in allied health, nursing, and pharmacology obtain initial training that leaves an important imprint on their future practice (Partnership for Solutions, 2002). In addition to the barriers of time constraints, oversight restrictions, resistance from the professions, and absence of political will, the overall health care financing system is a large impediment to integrating the core competencies into practice settings. Therefore, the committee believes steps must be taken to explore alternative ways of paying clinicians so as to foster such integration.

The lack of a supportive financial incentives structure becomes abundantly clear when one considers, for example, the kinds of services from which the chronically ill elderly would benefit and what Medicare fee-for-service pays for. Currently, Medicare fee-for-service does not generally pay for clinician time spent providing education that enables, for example, patients with diabetes and heart disease to make necessary lifestyle and behavioral changes, or for time spent helping such patients by teaching them how to actively manage their condition with the support of technology. Medicare fee-for-service also does not pay for the work involved in coordinating and integrating the various services such patients need across teams and settings (Institute of Medicine, 2002). Consequently, the financing system often undermines integration of the five competencies into practice, despite evidence that patients who are actively involved in managing and making decisions about their care have better quality and functional status outcomes at lower cost (Gifford et al., 1998; Superio-Cabuslay et al., 1996; Von Korff et al., 1998; Wagner et al., 2001).

As the largest payer, Medicare has a major effect on the system when it innovates (Institute of Medicine, 2002). Moreover, the committee believes that patients with chronic conditions—a sizable proportion of whom are covered by Medicare—would benefit greatly from integration of the five competencies into practice. There are a number of different options that could serve as models for these payment experiments, including capitation, bundled payments, bonuses, withholds, and various ways to share risk and responsibility between clinicians and payers (Bailit Health Purchasing, 2002; Guyatt et al., 2000). The committee encourages other payers to follow suit.

Recommendation 7: Through Medicare demonstration projects, the Centers for Medicare and Medicaid Services (CMS) should take the lead in funding experiments that will enable and create incentives for health professionals to integrate interdisciplinary approaches into educational or practice settings, with the goal of providing a training ground for students and clinicians that incorporates the five core competencies.

Research and Information

Along with oversight changes and supportive training environments, the committee believes that evidence of the efficacy of an educational intervention can be a catalyst for change. To this end, evidence related to the link between clinical education and health care quality needs to be better developed, as does evidence about various teaching approaches.

In a review of 117 trials in continuing education, fewer than 20 percent were found to use health care outcomes as their measure of effectiveness (Davis et al., 2000), and a review of 2,000 papers on continuing education showed that only about 5 percent assessed the relationship between course content and clinical outcomes (Jordan, 2000). Teaching itself is dominated by intuition and tradition, which do not always hold up when submitted to empirical verification (Tanenbaum, 1994; van der Vleuten et al., 2000). For example, studies have shown that lecture-based teaching of isolated

components, the most common means of imparting information in both academic and continuing education settings, fails in that it does not provide a way for students to integrate or apply the information provided (Wass et al., 2001).

Although there is significant public funding of health professions education, limited public and private resources are available for research that could help in determining whether the dollars are being well spent. In addition, much of the research that does exist is discipline-specific and therefore does not reflect the current practice environment.

The committee believes the time has come to focus energy and resources on developing a more robust and compelling evidence base about what educational content matters for patient care and what works in teaching clinicians so that educators, payers, and regulators can assess objectively what needs to be emphasized in the health professions curricula and what should be eliminated. The research should also span disciplines.

Recommendation 8: The Agency for Healthcare Research and Quality (AHRQ) and private foundations should support ongoing research projects addressing the five core competencies and their association with individual and population health, as well as research related to the link between the competencies and evidence-based education. Such projects should involve researchers across two or more disciplines.

The committee believes that incorporation of education-related measures into quality-reporting efforts and ongoing monitoring will be required to realize the vision articulated in this report. The lack of standardized information about the quality of clinical education makes the job of leaders seeking to reform such education more difficult. The lack of standardized measures also sets clinical education apart from the broader health care quality movement. A ranking—by NCQA regarding health plan quality or by *U.S. News and World Report* regarding hospitals, for example—forces leaders to focus their attention on improving performance on a given set of comparable metrics (National Committee for Quality Assurance, 2002; U.S. News and World Report, 2002). The National Healthcare Quality Report Card, anticipated for release by AHRQ in 2003 and annually thereafter, will likely further standardize quality measurement and focus attention on the strengths and weaknesses of the current system. Yet no education-related measures are anticipated for inclusion in this first annual report (Agency for Health Care Research Quality, 2002).

A focused effort to develop education-related measures must begin now, given the amount of time required to develop and test prospective measures before they can be incorporated into report cards. The committee recognizes that initially there will be a small number of measures ready for public reporting.

Recommendation 9: AHRQ should work with a representative group of health care leaders to develop measures reflecting the core set of competencies, set national goals for improvement, and issue a report to the public evaluating progress toward these goals. AHRQ should issue the first report, focused on clinical educational institutions, in 2005 and produce annual reports thereafter.

Providing Leadership

Significant reform in health professions education is a challenge to say the least. The oversight framework is a morass of different organizations with differing requirements and philosophies, now under considerable pressure to demonstrate greater accountability (Batalden et al., 2002; Finocchio et al., 1998; Leach, 2002; O'Neil and the Pew Health Professions

Commission, 1998). In academia, deans, department chairs, residency directors, and other leaders face a stream of requests for adding new elements to a curriculum that is already overcrowded. Shortages of key professionals, such as nurses and pharmacists, are another significant challenge. Moreover, funding for some academic health centers has been under pressure, and states are facing budget shortfalls that are causing them to trim education budgets, including funding for universities and community colleges (Griner and Danoff, 2000).

When change happens in health professions education, it does not happen overnight. Multiyear processes are required to develop, review, and achieve consensus on new requirements or methods before they can be implemented. Given this environment, the committee believes that reform of clinical education will be possible only with the skill and commitment of a broad range of health care leaders. A recent analysis and synthesis of 44 curriculum reform efforts revealed that leadership is the factor most often cited as affecting curriculum change (Bland et al., 2000).

Consequently, the committee believes that to maintain momentum for reform in clinical education, there will need to be biennial summits at which leaders who have demonstrated a real commitment to implementing the committee's overarching vision can gather. These summits should serve as a forum for leaders to take stock—including review of education-related performance measures and, over time, related trends against goals—and to define future plans. There should be a written report issued from the summit that captures such information and communicates it more broadly to the field.

Recommendation 10: Beginning in 2004, a biennial interdisciplinary summit should be held involving health care leaders in education, oversight processes, practice, and other areas. This summit

should focus on both reviewing progress against explicit targets and setting goals for the next phase with regard to the five competencies and other areas necessary to prepare professionals for the 21st-century health system.

Conclusion

The committee has set forth 10 major recommendations for reforming health professions education to enhance quality and meet the evolving needs of patients. Each of these recommendations focuses on ways of integrating a core set of competencies into health professions education. Taken together, they represent a mix of approaches related to oversight processes, the practice environment, research, public reporting, and leadership.

The staging of these recommendations is important. The first step is to articulate common terms so that shared definitions can inform interdisciplinary discussions about core competencies. Once the disciplines have agreed on a core set of competencies, public and private oversight bodies can consider how to incorporate such competencies into their processes—providing a catalyst for many educational institutions and professional associations, as well as support for those who have already moved toward adopting a competency-based approach. The committee believes that the development of common language and definition of core competencies should happen as rapidly as possible and by no later than 2004, given that the integration of core competencies into oversight processes will take considerable time, perhaps a decade or more if the efforts of ACGME and ACPE are any guide.

As the work of integrating core competencies into oversight processes proceeds, the efforts of leading practice organizations to integrate the core competencies into care delivery should be fostered through regional demonstration learning centers and Medicare demonstration projects. Simultaneously with these efforts, AHRQ and private foundations should provide support for research focused on the efficacy of the competencies and competency education and, most important, develop a set of measures reflecting the core set of competencies, along with national goals for improvement. Given that the committee calls upon AHRQ to issue a first report on health professions educational institutions by 2005, albeit with a limited number of initial measures, efforts related to reporting must begin immediately. Finally, the committee believes that biennial summits of health care leaders who control and shape education—starting in 2004—will be an important mechanism for integrating and furthering the efforts of those developing measures, practice and education innovators, researchers, and leaders from oversight organizations.

The committee is confident that its recommendations are both sound and feasible to implement because they are supported by a literature review, and informed by a broad range of leaders who shape education both directly and indirectly (see appendix C). Building a bridge to cross the quality chasm in health care cannot be done in isolation. The committee hopes that this report will jump start other efforts to reform clinical education, both individually and collectively, so that it focuses on continually reducing the burden of illness, injury, and disability, with the ultimate aim of improving the health status, functioning, and satisfaction of the American people (President's Advisory Commission on Consumer Protection and Quality in the Health Care Industry, 1998b). The public deserves nothing less.

References

ABIM Foundation. 2002. Medical professionalism in the new millennium: A physician charter. *Annals of Internal Medicine* 136 (3):243-46.

Accreditation Council for Graduate Medical Education. 1999. "General Competencies." Online. Available at http://www.acgme.org/outcome/comp/compFull.asp [accessed June,

2002].

Accreditation Council for Graduate Medical Education. 2002. "ACGME Outcome Project." Online. Available at http://www.acgme.org/outcome/about/faq.asp [accessed Aug. 27, 2002].

Agency for Healthcare Research and Quality. 2002. "NHQR Preliminary Measure Set." Online. Available at http://www.ahrq.gov/qual/nhqr02/nhqrprelim.htm [accessed Fall, 2002].

American Association of Medical Colleges. 1999. *Evidence Based Medicine Instruction* . Vol 2, No.3 edition Washington, DC: AAMC.

———. 2001. "Medical School Objectives Project." Online. Available at http://www.aamc.org/meded/msop/start.htm [accessed Sept., 2002].

American Board of Medical Specialties. 2000. *2000 ABMS Annual Report and Reference Handbook.*

American Council on Pharmaceutical Education. 2000. "Accreditation Manual-Ninth Addition ." Online. Available at www.acpe-accredit.org [accessed June, 2002].

———. 2002. "ACPE Web site." Online. Available at www.acpe.edu [accessed May 1, 2002].

American Nurses Association/NursingWorld.Org. 2001. "On-line Health and Safety Survey: Key Findings." Online. Available at http://nursingworld.org/surveys/keyfind.pdf [accessed 2002].

Bailit Health Purchasing. 2002. *Provider Incentive Models for Improving Quality of Care.* Washington, DC: National Health Care Purchasing Institute.

Baker, G.R., S. Gelmon, L. Headrick, M. Knapp, L. Norman, D. Quinn, and D. Neuhauser. 1998. Collaborating for improvement in health professions education. *Quality Management in Health Care* 6 (2):1-11.

Bashook, P.G., S.H. Miller, J. Parboosingh, and S.D. Horowitz. 2000. "Credentialing Physician Specialists: A World Perspective." Online. Available at http://www.abms.org/Downloads/Conferences/Credentialing%20Physician%20Specialists.pdf [accessed Sept. 15, 2002].

Batalden, P., D. Leach, S. Swing, H. Dreyfus, and S. Dreyfus. 2002. General competencies and accreditation in graduate medical education. *Health Affairs* 21 (5):103-11.

Bellack, J.P., and E.H. O'Neil. 2000. Recreating nursing practice for a new century: Recommendations and implications of the pew health professions commissions final report. *Nursing & Health Care Perspectives* 21 (1):14-21.

Bland, C.J., S. Starnaman, L. Wersal, L. Moorhead-Rosenberg, S. Zonia, and R. Henry. 2000. Curricular change in medical schools: How to succeed. *Academic Medicine* 75 (6):575-94.

Board of Pharmaceutical Specialties. 2002. "Recertification." Online. Available at http://www.bpsweb.org/BPS/recert-gen.html#top [accessed Sept., 2002].

Brady, M., J.D. Leuner, J.P. Bellack, R.S. Loquist, P. F. Cipriano, and E.H. O'Neil. 2001. A proposed framework for differentiating the 21 pew competencies by level of nursing education. *Nursing & Health Care Perspectives* 22 (1):30-35.

Buerhaus, P.I., and L. Norman. 2001. Its time to require theory and methods of quality improvement in basic and graduate nursing education. *Nursing Outlook* 49 (2):67-69.

Byrd, G. 2002. Can the profession of pharmacy serve as a model for health informationist professionals? *Journal of Medical Library Association* 90 (1):68-75.

Calabretta, N. 2002. Consumer-driven, patient-centered health care in the age of electronic information. *Journal of Medical Library Association* 90 (1):32-37.

Cantillon, P., and R. Jones. 1999. Does continuing medical education in general practice make a difference? *British Medical Journal* 318 (7193):1276-79.

Carraccio, C., S.D. Wolfsthal, R. Englander, K. Ferentz, and C. Martin. 2002. Shifting paradigms: From flexner to competencies. *Academic Medicine* 77 (5):361-67.

Center for the Advancement of Pharmaceutical Education [CAPE] Advisory Panel on Educational Outcomes. 1998. "Educational Outcomes." Online. Available at http://www.aacp.org/Docs/MainNavigation/Resources/3933_edoutcom.doc?DocTypeID=4&TrackID=&VID=1&CID=410&DID=366 [accessed Dec. 10, 2002].

Chassin, M.R., R.W. Galvin, and the National

Roundtable on Health Care Quality. 1998. The urgent need to improve health care quality. *Journal of the American Medical Association* 280 (11):1000-1005.

Christakis, N.A. 1995. The similarity and frequency of proposals to reform U.S. medical education: Constant concerns. *Journal of American Medical Association* 274 (9):706-11.

Collier, S. March 2002. Workforce Shortages. Personal communication to Ann Greiner.

Commission on Collegiate Nursing Education. 2002. "CCNE Accreditation." Online. Available at http://www.aacn.nche.edu/Accreditation/ [accessed 2002].

Council on Graduate Medical Education. 1999. *Physician Education for a Changing Health Care Environment*. Rockville, MD: Health Resources and Services Administration.

Counsell, S., R. Kennedy, P. Szwabo, N. Wadsworth, and C. Wohlgemuth. 1999. Curriculum recommendations for resident training in geriatrics interdisciplinary team care. *Journal of the American Geriatrics Society* 47 (9):1145-48.

Davis, D., M.A. OBrien, N. Freemantle, F.M. Wolf, P. Mazmanian, and A. Taylor-Vaisey. 1999. Impact of formal continuing medical education: Do conferences, workshops, rounds, and other traditional continuing education activities change physician behavior or health care outcomes? *Journal of American Medical Association* 282 (9):867-74.

Davis, D., M.A. Thomson O'Brien, and N. Freemantle. 2000. Review: Interactive, but not didactic, continuing medical education is effective in changing physician performance. *Database of Abstracts of Reviews of Effectiveness* Volume 132 (2):75.

Detmer, D.E. 1997. Knowledge: A mountain or a stream? *Science* 275 (5308):1859.

Epstein, R.M., and E.M. Hundert. 2002. Defining and assessing professional competence. *Journal of the American Medical Association* 287 (2):226-35.

Federation of State Medical Boards. 2002. "Post-Licensure Assessment System." Online. Available at http://www.fsmb.org/PLASmain. htm [accessed Aug., 2002].

Ferrill, M.J., L.L. Norton, and S.J. Blalock. 1999. Determining the statistical knowledge of pharmacy practitioners: A survey and review of the literature. *American Journal of Pharmaceutical Education* 63 (3)

Finocchio, L. J., C. M. Dower, N. T. Blick, C. M. Gragnola, and the Taskforce on Health Care Workforce Regulation. 1998. *Strengthening Consumer Protection: Priorities for Health Care Workforce Regulation*. San Francisco, CA: Pew Health Professions Commission.

Frosch, D.L., and R.M. Kaplan. 1999. Shared decision making in clinical medicine: Past research and future directions. *American Journal of Preventive Medicine* 17 (4):285-94.

Gerteis, M., S. Edgman-Levitan, J. Daley, and T. Delbanco, editors. 1993. *Through the Patient Eyes*. Vol. San Francisco, CA: Josey-Bass.

Gifford, A.L., D.D. Laurent, V.M. Gonzales, et al. 1998. Pilot randomized trial of education to improve self-management skills of men with symptomatic HIV/AIDS. *Journal of Acquired Immune Deficiency Syndromes and Human Retrovirology* 18 (2):136-44.

Gorman, P.J.M., A.H.M. Meier, C. Rawn, and T.M. M. Krummel. 2000. The future of medical education is no longer blood and guts, it is bits and bytes. *American Journal of Surgery* 180 (5):353-56.

Grantmakers in Health. 2001. *Training the Health Worklforce of Tommorow*. Washington, DC: Grantmakers In Health .

Green, M.L. 2000. Evidence-based medicine training in internal medicine residency programs a national survey. *Journal of General Internal Medicine* 15 (2):129-33.

Griner, P.F.M., and D.M. Danoff. 2000. Sustaining change in medical education. *Journal of American Medical Association* 283 (18):2429-31.

Guyatt, G. 1992. Evidence-based medicine. A new approach to teaching the practice of medicine. Evidence-Based Medicine Working Group. *Journal of American Medical Association* 268 (17):2420-2425.

Guyatt, G.H., R.B. Haynes, R.Z. Jaeschke, D.J. Cook, L. Green, C.D. Naylor, M. Wilson, and W.S. Richardson. 2000. Users guide to the medical literature: XXV. Evidence-based medicine: Principles for applying the users guides to patient care. *Journal of American Medical Association* 284 (10):1290-1296.

Hafferty, F. 1998. Beyond curriculum reform: confronting medicine's hidden curriculum. *Academic Medicine* 73 (4):403-7.

Halpern, J. 1996. The measurement of quality of care in the veterans health administration. *Medical Care* 34 (3):55-68.

Halpern, R., M.Y. Lee, P.R. Boulter, and R.R. Phillips. 2001. A synthesis of nine major reports on physicians competencies for the emerging practice environment. *Academic Medicine* 76 (6):606-15.

Harden, R.M. 2002. Developments in outcome-based education. *Medical Teacher* 24 (2):117-20.

Harmening, D.M. 1999. "Pioneering Allied Health Clinical Education Reform. A National Consensus Conference." Online. Available at ftp://ftp.hrsa.gov/bhpr/publications/cerpdf.pdf [accessed Aug., 2002].

Health Resources and Services Administration. 1999. *Building the Future of Allied Health: Report of the Implementation Task Force of the National Commission on Allied Health.* Rockville, MD: Health Resources and Services Administration.

Hovenga, E.J. 2000. Global health informatics education. *Studies in Health Technology & Informatics* 57:3-14.

Hundert, E.M., F. Hafferty, and D. Christakis. 1996. Characteristics of the informal curriculum and trainees ethical choices. *Academic Medicine* 71 (6):624-42.

Hyde, R.S., and J.M. Vermillion. 1996. Driving quality through Hoshin planning. *Joint Commission Journal on Quality Improvement* 22 (1):27-35.

Ingersoll, G. 2000. Evidence-based nursing: What it is and what it isnt. *Nursing Outlook* 48:151-52.

Institute of Medicine. 2000. *To Err Is Human: Building a Safer Health System.* Linda T. Kohn, Janet M. Corrigan, and Molla S. Donaldson, eds. Washington, DC: National Academy Press.

———. 2001. *Crossing the Quality Chasm: A New Health System for the 21st Century.*

Washington, DC: National Academy Press.

Institute of Medicine. 2002. *Leadership By Example.* Washington, DC: National Academies Press.

Jablonover, R.S., D.J. Blackman, E.B. Bass, G. Morrison, and A.H. Goroll. 2000. Evaluation of a national curriculum reform effort for the medicine core clerkship. *Journal of General Internal Medicine* 15 (7): 484-91.

Jordan, S. 2000. Educational input and patient outcomes: Exploring the gap. *Journal of Advanced Nursing* 31 (2):461-71.

Lavin, M.A., I. Ruebling, R. Banks, L. Block, M. Counte, G. Furman, P. Miller, C. Reese , V. Viehmann, and J. Holt. 2001. Interdisciplinary health professional education: A historical review. *Advances in Health Sciences Education* 6 (1):25-47.

Leach, D.C. 2002. Building and assessing competence: the potential for evidence-based graduate medical education. *Qual Manag Health Care* 11(1):39-44.

Leach, D.C. 2002. Competence is a habit. *Journal of the American Medical Association* 287 (2):243-44.

Lenburg, C., R. Redman, and P. Hinton. 1999. "Competency Assessment: Methods for Development and Implementation in Nursing Education." Online. [accessed Mar. 19, 2002].

Mansell, D., R.M. Poses, L. Kazis, and C.A. Duefield. 2000. Clinical factors that influence patients desire for participation in decisions about illness. *Archives of Medicine* 160:2991-96.

Marwick, C. 2000. Will evidence-based practice help span gulf between medicine and law? *Journal of American Medical Association* 283 (21):2775-76.

Maudsley, G. 2001. What issues are raised by evaluating problem-based undergraduate medical curricula? Making healthy connections across the literature. [Review] [93 refs]. *Journal of Evaluation in Clinical Practice* 7 (3):311-24.

Mazur, D.J. and D.H. Hickam. 1997. Patients preferences for risk disclosure and role in decision making for invasive medical procedures . *Journal of General Internal Medicine* 12:114-17.

Mazurek, B. 2002. Strategies for overcoming barriers in implementing evidence-based practice. *Periatric Nursing* 28 (2):159-61.

Mitchell, G. 1999. Evidence-based practice: Critique and alternative view. *Nursing Science Quarterly* Vol. 12, No. 1:30-35.

Murray, E., L. Gruppen, P. Catton, R. Hays, and J.O. Woolliscroft. 2000. The accountability of clinical education: Its definition and assessment. *Medical Education* 34 (10):871-79.

National Association of Boards of Pharmacy. 2002. "Examinations -- NAPLEX." Online. Available at http://www.nabp.net/ [accessed Aug. 10, 2002].

National Committee for Quality Assurance. 2002. "What Does NCQA Review When It Accredits an HMO?" Online. Available at http://www. ncqa.org/Programs/Accreditation/MCO/ mcostdsoverview.htm [accessed 2002].

National Council of State Boards of Nursing. 2001. "NCLEX - RN@ Examination: Test Plan for the National Council Licensure Examination for Registered Nurses." Online. Available at http:// www.ncsbn.org/public/testing/res/ NCSBNRNTestPlanBooklet.pdf [accessed Aug., 2002].

National Council of State Boards of Nursing, I. 1997-2000. "Nursing Regulation: Examination Pass Rates & Licensure Statistics." Online. Available at http://www.ncsbn.org/public/ regulation/licensure_stats.htm [accessed 2002].

National League for Nursing Accrediting Commission. 2002. "National League for Nursing Accreditation Commission Website ." Online. Available at www.nlnac.org [accessed May 31, 2002].

OBrien, T., N. Freemantle, A.D. Oxman, F. Wolf, D. A. Davis, and J. Herrin. 2001. Continuing education meetings and workshops: Effects on professional practice and health care outcomes. *Cochrane Database System Review* (2): CD003030.

OConnor, G.T., S.K. Plume, E.M. Olmstead, J.R. Morton, C.T. Maloney, W.C. Nugent, F. Hernandez, Jr. , R. Clough, B.J. Leavitt, L.H. Coffin, C.A. Marrin, D. Wennberg, J.D. Birkmeyer, D.C. Charlesworth, D.J. Malenka, H.B. Quinton, and J.F. Kasper. 1996. A regional intervention to improve the hospital mortality associated with coronary artery bypass graft surgery. The Northern New England Cardiovascular Disease Study Group. *Journal of the American Medical Association* 275 (11):841-46.

ONeil, E. H. and the Pew Health Professions Commission. 1998. *Recreating health professional practice for a new century - The fourth report of the PEW health professions Commission.* San Francisco, CA: Pew Health Professions Commission.

Partnership for Solutions. 2002. "Physician Concerns: Caring for People with Chronic Conditions." Online. Available at http://www. partnershipforsolutions.org/pdf_files/2002/ physicianccern.pdf [accessed Oct. 8, 2002].

Pew Health Professions Commission. 1995. *Critical Challenges: Revitalizing the Health Professions for the Twenty-First Century.* San Francisco, CA: UCSF Center for the Health Professions:

Phillips, R.L. Jr, D.C. Harper, M. Wakefield, L.A. Green, and G.E. Fryer, Jr. 2002. Can nurse practitioners and physicians beat parochialism into plowshares? *Health Affairs* 21 (5):133-42.

Platt, D., and C. Laird. 1995. CQI: Using the Hoshin planning system to design an orientation process. *Radiology Management* 17 (2):42-50.

Pomeroy, W.M., and I. Philp. 1994. Healthcare teams: An interdisciplinary workshop for undergraduates. *Medical Teacher*:6p.

President's Advisory Commission on Consumer Protection and Quality in the Health Care Industry. 1998. "Quality First: Better Health Care for All Americans." Online. Available at http://www.hcqualitycommission.gov/final/ [accessed Sept. 9, 2000].

Satya-Murti, S. 2000. Evidence-based clinical practice: Concepts and approaches. *The Journal of American Medical Association* 282 (17):2306-7.

Schuster, M.A., E.A. McGlynn, and R.H. Brook. 1998. How good is the quality of health care in the United States? *Milbank Quarterly* 76 (4):517-63, 509.

Shell, R. 2001. Perceived barriers to teaching for critical thinking by BSN nursing faculty. *Nursing & Health Care Perspectives* 22 (6):286-91.

Superio-Cabuslay, E., M.M. Ward, and K.R. Lorig. 1996. Patient education interventions in osteoarthritis and rheumatoid arthritis: A meta-analytic comparison with nonsteroidal anti-inflammatory drug treatment. *Arthritis Care Research* 9 (4):292-301.

Swankin, D. 30 May 2002a . Continuing Competence. Personal communication to Elisa Knebel.

Swankin, D.S. 2002b. *Results of a Survey of Selected State Health Licensing Boards and Health Voluntary Certification Agencies Concerning their Continuing Competence Programs and Requirements.* Washington, DC: Citizen Advocacy Center.

Tanenbaum, S.J. 1994. Knowing and acting in medical practice: the epistemological politics of outcomes research. *J Health Polit Policy Law* 19 (1):27-44.

U.S. News and World Report. "Latest Hospital Rankings." Online. Available at www.usnews. com/usnews/nycu/health/hosptl/tophosp.htm [accessed Summer, 2002].

United States Medical Licensing Exam. 2002. "United States Medical Licensing Examination - Steps 1, 2, 3." Online. Available at http://www. usmle.org/step1/intro.htm [accessed Aug. 10, 2002].

van der Vleuten, C.M., D.M. Dolmans, and A.A. Scherpbier. 2000. The need for evidence in education. *Medical Teacher* 22 (3):246-50.

Von Korff, M., J.E. Moore, K.R. Lorig, et al. 1998. A randomized trial of a lay person-led self-management group intervention for back pain patients in primary care. *Spine* 23 (23):2608-51.

Wagner, E.H., R.E. Glasgow, C. Davis, A.E. Bonomi, L. Provost, D. McCulloch, P. Carver, and C. Sixta. 2001. Quality improvement in chronic illness care: A collaborative approach. *Joint Commission Journal on Quality Improvement* 27 (2):63-80.

Wass, V., C. Van der Vleuten, J. Shatzer, and R. Jones. 2001. Assessment of clinical competence. *Lancet* 357 (9260):945-49.

Weed, L.L. and L. Weed. 1999. Opening the black box of clinical judgment. Part II: consumer protection and the patients role. *British Medical Journal.* November 13

Wennberg, J.H. 1998. *The Dartmouth Atlas of Health Care 1998.* Hanover, NH: Center for the Evaluation Clinical Sciences, Dartmouth University.

Woolf, S.H. 2000. Taking critical appraisal to extremes: The need for balance in the evaluation of evidence. *Journal of Family Practice* 49 (12):1081-85.

Wu, S., and A. Green. 2000. *Projection of Chronic Illness Prevalence and Cost Inflation.* California: RAND Health.

Yoder-Wise, P.S. 2002. State and association/certifying boards: CE requirements. *Journal of Continuing Education in Nursing* 33 (1):3-11.

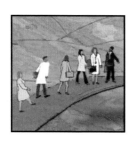

Chapter 1
Introduction

Many organizations, experts, health professionals, and, increasingly, the American public question whether quality health care can be delivered under the existing health care system, noting that health care today harms too frequently and consistently fails to deliver its potential benefits (Blendon et al., 2001; Kaiser Family Foundation and Agency for Healthcare Research and Quality, 2000; Wirthlin Worldwide, 2001). Studies by expert bodies first documented the serious and pervasive nature of the quality problem with reports of overuse of services, such as excessive prescribing of antibiotics to children; misuse of services, such as incorrect dosages of drugs being administered to patients; and underuse of services, such as not employing effective prevention strategies with patients (Chassin, 1998; President's Advisory Commission on Consumer Protection and Quality in the Health Care Industry, 1998; Schuster et al., 1998). Such errors, as documented by the authors of *To Err Is Human: Building a Safer Health System*, result in tens of thousands of Americans dying each year and hundreds of thousands suffering or being sick (Institute of Medicine, 2000).

In the report *Crossing the Quality Chasm: A New Health System for the 21st Century* (Institute of Medicine, 2001) the same Institute of Medicine (IOM) committee that authored *To Err Is Human* emphasizes that such safety problems occur because of the system's inability to translate knowledge into practice, to apply new technology safely and appropriately, and to make best use of its resources—both financial and human. In the face of these system failures, the *Quality Chasm* report stresses that the rapidly increasing chronic care population only compounds the need for a redesigned health system. Fully 40 percent of the U.S. population—125 million Americans—live with some type of chronic condition, and about half of them live with multiple such conditions (Wu and Green, 2000).

The *Quality Chasm* report also emphasizes that blaming health providers or asking them to just try harder is not the answer to addressing the health care system's current flaws and future challenges. Gaps in quality are occurring in the hands of health professionals highly dedicated to doing a good job, but working within a system that does not support them in achieving what they want and ought to be providing for patients. The *Quality Chasm* report sets forth an ambitious agenda for the redesign of this broken health care system. First, the system must be designed to provide care that achieves six national quality aims: safety, effectiveness, patient-centeredness, timeliness, efficiency, and equity. The system must serve the needs of patients, ensuring that they are fully informed, retain control, participate in care delivery whenever possible, and receive care that is respectful of their values and preferences. Moreover, the system must facilitate the application of scientific knowledge to practice by providing clinicians with the tools and support necessary to deliver evidence-based care consistently and safely.

Implementing this agenda has important implications for current and future health professionals. Such changes mean that health professionals need to be better prepared. They must be educated, trained, and regulated differently so they can function as effectively as possible in a reformed health system, a system founded on enhanced quality and safety as envisioned in the *Quality Chasm* report.

Origins of the Study

The *Quality Chasm* report emphasizes the need for additional study to understand the effects of the recommended changes on how the workforce is educated for practice, how it is deployed, and how it is held accountable. One recommendation of the report is that a multidisciplinary summit of leaders within the health professions be held to discuss and develop strategies for restructuring clinical education to be consistent with the six national quality aims outlined above across the continuum of education for the allied health, medical, nursing, and pharmacy professions.

In 2001, the Health Resources and Services Administration (HRSA) within the Department of Health and Human Services (DHHS) asked the IOM's Board on Health Care Services to convene a committee that would be charged with coordinating the recommended summit and drafting a follow-up report. The Committee on the Health Professions Education Summit was formed for this purpose. The committee included members with expertise and experience in academic and continuing allied health, medical, nursing, and pharmacy education; multidisciplinary clinical training; health professions licensure and oversight processes; professional credentialing; and health care delivery and quality.

Health Professions Education Summit

Summit Planning

The committee held three meetings during 2002—a planning meeting to review the literature and prepare for the summit, a meeting during the summit to identify major objectives for reform that would inform the specific actions proposed by participants, and a post-summit meeting. At this last meeting, the committee reviewed a draft of this report and its recommendations.

In preparation for the summit, the committee reviewed the new or enhanced skills required by health professionals to function in the changing health care environment as cited in the *Quality Chasm* report (Chapter 9). (See Chapter 3 for a more in-depth discussion.) The committee grouped those skills and defined five overarching competencies needed by today's health care professionals: provide patient-centered care, work in interdisciplinary teams, employ evidence-based practice, apply quality improvement approaches, and utilize informatics.

The committee then examined the extent to which students and practicing health professionals were required to receive education in these areas. To perform this examination, the committee worked with IOM staff on papers that surveyed the published literature and existing requirements and standards promulgated by the accrediting and licensing bodies of various health professions, consulted with experts in clinical education, and gathered input from other interested organizations. An examination of available evaluation data provided insight into what is and is not working, as well as the limitations of education efforts to date. Background papers on each of the five competencies were provided to summit participants.

The committee endeavored to make the most of the evidence and substantial experience available, but found in its review of the available literature, consultation with experts, and input from other interested parties that the evidence base needed to assess the current status of education and oversight processes of the health professions in each of the five competencies is limited. There have been few rigorous long-term evaluations of any aspect of health professions education, much less evaluations related to the five competencies (Furze and Pearcey, 1999; Murray et al., 2000). It is difficult to locate even a single evaluation that measures changes in patient outcomes or satisfaction as a result of any revision of curriculum. Most studies of clinical education are qualitative, employing anecdotal observation of student performance or self-assessments by learners of changes in knowledge, skills, and attitudes For the quantitative studies available, less-rigorous evaluation measures, such as student satisfaction, are often employed (Belfield et al., 2001; Cooper et al., 2001; Jordan, 2000; O'Brien et al., 2001). The majority of documented experiences come from medicine, fewer from nursing and pharmacy, and very few from allied health (Department of Health and Human Services, 1998).

In planning the summit and identifying a list of participants, the committee sought input from the Council on Graduate Medical Education and the National Advisory Council on Nurse

Education and Practice, advisory committees to HSRA. They provided input that led to the summit participants' encompassing a multidisciplinary group of allied health, nursing, medical, and pharmacy educators and students; health industry representatives; regulators and accreditors; health organization representatives; consumers; and policy leaders. Care was taken to include professionals from diverse occupations. Individuals from other key organizations also were consulted during the planning process. The names and affiliations of the more than 150 attendees are listed in Appendix D.

Summit Execution

The summit began with plenary sessions led by noted health experts, including Kenneth Shine, then president of the IOM; William Richardson, president of the W. K. Kellogg Foundation; and Donald M. Berwick, president of the Institute for Healthcare Improvement. These sessions were designed to set the context of the current reality of health professions education and the new health care environment that future health professionals must be educated to address. Included was a panel discussion on educational implications of caring for the chronically ill. The full summit agenda is provided in Appendix B.

Following the plenary sessions, participants worked in small interdisciplinary groups to draft proposed strategies for integrating one of the above five competencies into clinical education (see Box 1-1). The committee then reviewed and synthesized these strategies and, using prioritization tools, chose seven priority strategies for the reform of health professions education on which summit participants focused for the next day. On day two of the summit, participants drafted actions to advance these strategies for reform. The main strategies, aggregated into five groups, are detailed in Appendix C.

Box 1-1. Facilitating the Summit

Expert facilitators used the Hoshin method, a strategic planning method developed in Japan, as well as other creative problem-solving tools, to facilitate the strategy generation process (Counsell et al., 1999; Hyde and Vermillion, 1996; Platt and Laird, 1995).

On day one of the summit, each participant, using a tool called *brainwriting*, generated a list of strategies for integration of the five competencies into health professions education. Then in small groups, participants used *affinity diagrams* to arrange the more than 1700 strategies that had been generated into common groupings of overarching strategies. Using another tool, the *interrelationship digraph*, the groups were then able to identify the main drivers for reform among these overarching strategies.

The committee convened on the evening of day one of the summit to review and synthesize these strategies. Using the identified drivers for reform and the rest of the data from day one, the committee applied prioritization tools to select seven overarching strategies for the reform of health professions education.

During day two, participants selected one of these strategies on which they felt they could make the most significant contribution. Working again in small, self-selected, interdisciplinary groups, participants used a tool called a *tree diagram* to develop individual actions, with related achievable measures, that they would take over the next 1 to 3 years to make their contribution.

Post-Summit Activities

The committee's final meeting was held to review a draft of this report and its recommendations. This review was based on an examination of the salient literature, as well as consideration of the strategies and actions proposed at the summit.

Scope of the Report

The content of this report reflects the committee's commitment to carrying out its stated charge. Although a number of important and often controversial areas were discussed during the committee's deliberations and are briefly mentioned in the report, recommendations related to those issues falling outside the scope of the committee's charge are not addressed. These issues include the distribution, composition, and shortages of the health care workforce; issues related to education preparation and entry into practice;

the financing of health professions education;[1] changing skill requirements for new occupations; and student recruitment and admissions policies. These issues remain important, and the committee hopes this report will influence or shape deliberations in these other areas.

Building Upon Previous Reform Efforts

In carrying out its charge, the committee was cognizant of the many outstanding efforts that have been made to articulate a vision for the reform of health professions education (Bellack and O'Neil, 2000; Council on Graduate Medical Education, 1999; Halpern et al., 2001; Harmening, 1999; Hegge, 1995; Long, 1994; Mennin, 1998; O'Neil and the Pew Health Professions Commission, 1998). There has been no shortage of good ideas on how to reform clinical education, the striking feature of these ideas being their similarity with regard to

---

[1] A current Institute of Medicine study addressing academic health centers is considering financing questions.

the problems identified and proposed solutions (Bellack and O'Neil, 2000; Christakis, 1995; Enarson and Burg, 1992; Rivo et al., 1993).

Unfortunately, reform of health professions education can be exceedingly slow and difficult to accomplish. A number of reasons have been cited for the lack of reform. Health professions education frequently occurs in an environment of separately housed professional schools and separate clinical arenas governed by separate deans, directors, and department chairs, often resulting in the protection of specific specialties or interests at the cost of the educational goals of the school (Enarson and Burg, 1992; Regan-Smith, 1998). Another reason is the financing of academic centers which has resulted in many institutions valuing research and clinical activities at the expense of education (Ludmerer, 1999; Regan-Smith, 1998). This complex web of competing educational and oversight systems and processes has made it difficult for successful institution- or classroom-based innovations to diffuse on a widespread basis. Many reform efforts have also not taken root among the professions because there has been little motivation to change and a lack of the leadership needed to carry the reforms forward. This lack of motivation and leadership in turn reflects the absence of a clear understanding of why such changes would be any better than current practice or how they could be accomplished comprehensively. Finally, coordination and collaboration within and among the professions has been extremely difficult to achieve, and this has posed a key barrier to reform.

For these reasons, the committee believes a more intense and coordinated effort will be needed that spans the various health professions and those entities responsible for shaping education in each field. The committee believes the time is ripe to build upon previous reform efforts, galvanizing the education, practice, and oversight communities.

First, these groups increasingly understand the extent of quality problems and recognize that the system needs wholesale restructuring; an essential aspect of that restructuring is

reform of the content, skills, and values taught to students and faculty. In a 2001 survey of more than 1,000 health care professionals, 58 percent of providers and administrators rated health care in the United States as not very good, and 4 of 5 respondents said they believed fundamental changes are needed in the U.S. health care system (Wirthlin Worldwide, 2001). In another survey, more than half of physicians said they believe their ability to deliver quality care has decreased in the past 5 years (Blendon et al., 2001). Second, health professionals are dissatisfied with their working and training conditions, and recruitment difficulties and personnel shortages have become pressing issues (Hart et al., 2002; Sochalski, 2002). This dissatisfaction is driven in part by the mismatch between what health professionals are called upon to do and what they are educated to do (Blumenthal et al., 2001; Cantor et al., 1993; Weissman et al., 2001). Indeed, two-thirds of physicians in a recent study reported that their training was inadequate to enable them to coordinate care for patients or educate patients with chronic conditions (Partnership for Solutions, 2002). Finally, the health care industry has identified shortcomings of recent graduates, stating that an increasing amount of time and resources must be spent to teach new professionals the competencies required in today's workplace (Institute of Medicine, 2000; National Council for State Boards of Nursing, 2001). Change is needed at all levels, including, among others, the culture and values of educational institutions, the infrastructures in which professions are educated, curricula and teaching methods, the standards and guidelines governing education, the ways in which faculty are prepared and rewarded, and the leadership in schools and oversight organizations.

Definitional Issues

To address health professions education, it is necessary to clarify several key terms. To this end, the committee established common descriptions and terms for the key entities and concepts involved in its work, as described below.

Health Professions

This report places special emphasis on the following health professionals: nurses (both registered and advanced practice), pharmacists, physician assistants, physicians, and others that sometime come under the rubric of *allied health*. However, the observations, conclusions, and recommendations in this report will be of value to all health professionals caring for patients, including, for example, psychologists, counselors, and social workers. The committee acknowledges that defining what is meant by the term *allied health* and specifying the disciplines it encompasses is problematic. Understandably, many of the disciplines wish to avoid being categorized under such a catch-all term. When possible, therefore, this report refers to health professionals by their specific names (e.g., occupational therapists or dental hygienists). In some cases, however, when brevity is of concern, the committee employs the term *allied health* to refer to the 10 fields recognized by the IOM's Committee to Study the Role of Allied Health Personnel (Institute of Medicine, 1989) as the largest and best known: clinical laboratory technology, dental services, dietetic services, emergency medical services, medical records/health information management, occupational therapy, physical therapy, radiological services, respiratory therapy, and speech–language pathology/audiology. Yet it must be recognized that these disciplines vary greatly in the amount and level of education required, the nature of clinical involvement, and the ability to practice independently as opposed to working only under the direct supervision of others.

Education, Competency, and Oversight

The term *education* as used in this report refers to formal efforts to provide information and experience and develop new skills and competencies among students or practicing health professionals. *Continuing education* refers to organized educational activities undertaken by health professionals who have graduated from their respective degree programs and are already in professional practice. *Faculty* comprise the teaching staff and members of the administrative staff having academic rank in an educational institution, and include clinician teachers and residents.

Currently there is no agreed-upon definition of *competency* in health professions education. For the purposes of this report, the committee defines *professional competence* as the habitual and judicious use of communication, knowledge, technical skills, clinical reasoning, emotions, values, and reflection in daily practice for the benefit of the individuals and community being served (Hundert et al., 1996). *Competency-based education* refers to educational programs designed to ensure that students achieve prespecified levels of competence in a given field or training activity. A *core competency* is the identified knowledge, ability, or expertise in a specific subject area or skill set that is shared across the health professions. In this report, competency denotes an individual clinician's actual performance in a specific job function or task, and competencies or competency areas are skills considered necessary to perform a specific job or service (Kelly-Thomas, 1998).

The term *oversight processes* denotes the array of mechanisms and rules meant to ensure that health professionals are properly educated and competent to practice. It encompasses accreditation of educational programs serving health professionals, as well as professional licensure and certification. The spectrum of oversight processes can also include organizational accreditation, which serves to accredit practice institutions and health plans, but has some impact on the continuing competence of practicing professionals as well through the standards imposed.

Organization of the Report

This report offers a vision of a better-prepared health workforce and specific strategies, actions, and related recommendations for achieving that vision. Specifically, the report provides:

- Discussion of the challenges facing the reform of the health system and their implications for health professions education (Chapter 2).

- Explication of the core competencies needed by health professionals to be effective in the 21st-century health system (Chapter 3).

- Assessment of the extent to which the committee's vision is currently addressed by academic education programs among selected health professions (Chapter 4).

- Assessment of the extent to which this vision is currently addressed by licensure, accreditation, and certification bodies of selected health professions (Chapter 5).

- Recommendations developed by the committee for the reform of clinical education (Chapter 6)

The committee's conclusions and recommendations in these areas are presented in the respective chapters, highlighted in bold print. The appendices contain more-detailed information about the summit, a list of participants, and strategies and actions proposed by summit participants. It was not possible to present the over 200 actions identified by the summit participants in the report, but those at the national level and a small number at the institutional level are included.

References

Belfield, C., H. Thomas, A. Bullock, R. Eynon, and D. Wall. 2001. Measuring effectiveness for best evidence medical education: A discussion. *Medical Teacher* 23 (2):164-70.

Bellack, J.P., and E.H. O'Neil. 2000. Recreating nursing practice for a new century: Recommendations and implications of the PEW health professions commissions final report. *Nursing & Health Care Perspectives* 21 (1):14-21.

Blendon, R.J., C. Schoen, K. Donelan, R. Osborn, C. M. DesRoches, K. Scoles, K. Davis, K. Binns, and K. Zapert. 2001. Physicians views on quality of care: A five-country comparison. *Health Affairs* 20 (3):233-43.

Blumenthal, D., M. Gokhale, E.G. Campbell, and J. S. Weissman. 2001. Preparedness for clinical practice: Reports of graduating residents at academic health centers. *Journal of the American Medical Association* 286 (9):1027-34.

Cantor, J.C., L.C. Baker, and R.G. Hughes. 1993. Preparedness for practice. Young physicians views of their professional education. *JAMA* 270 (9):1035-40.

Chassin, M.R. 1998. Is health care ready for Six Sigma quality? *Milbank Quarterly* 76 (4):565-91, 510.

Christakis, N.A. 1995. The similarity and frequency of proposals to reform U.S. medical education: Constant concerns. *Journal of American Medical Association* 274 (9):706-11.

Cooper, H., C. Carlisle, T. Gibbs, and C. Watkins. 2001. Developing an evidence base for interdisciplinary learning: A systematic review. *Journal of Advanced Nursing* 35 (2):228-37.

Council on Graduate Medical Education. 1999. *Physician Education for a Changing Health Care Environment*. Rockville, MD: Health Resources and Services Administration.

Counsell, S., R. Kennedy, P. Szwabo, N. Wadsworth, and C. Wohlgemuth. 1999. Curriculum recommendations for resident training in geriatrics interdisciplinary team care. *Journal of the American Geriatrics Society* 47 (9):1145-48.

Department of Health and Human Services, Health Resources and Services Administration, Bureau of Primary Health Care. 1998. Health Center Program Expectations. *Bureau of Primary Health Care Policy Information Notice: 98-23*.

Enarson, C., and F.D. Burg. 1992. An overview of reform initiatives in medical education. 1906 through 1992. [Review] [22 refs]. *Journal of American Medical Association* 268 (9):1141-43.

Furze, G. and P. Pearcey. 1999. Continuing education in nursing: a review of the literature. *Journal of Advanced Nursing* 29 (2)

Halpern, R., M.Y. Lee, P.R. Boulter, and R.R. Phillips. 2001. A synthesis of nine major reports on physicians competencies for the emerging practice environment. *Academic Medicine* 76 (6):606-15.

Harmening, D.M. 1999. "Pioneering Allied Health Clinical Education Reform. A National Consensus Conference." Online. Available at ftp://ftp.hrsa.gov/bhpr/publications/cerpdf.pdf [accessed Aug., 2002].

Hart, L.G., E. Salsberg, D.M. Phillips, and D.M. Lishner. 2002. Rural health care providers in the United States. *Journal of Rural Health* 18 Suppl:211-32.

Hegge, M. 1995. Restructuring registered nurse curricula. [Review] [41 refs]. *Nurse Educator* 20 (6):39-44.

Hundert, E.M., F. Hafferty, and D. Christakis. 1996. Characteristics of the informal curriculum and trainees ethical choices. *Academic Medicine* 71 (6):624-42.

Hyde, R.S., and J.M. Vermillion. 1996. Driving quality through Hoshin planning. *Joint Commission Journal on Quality Improvement* 22 (1):27-35.

Institute of Medicine. 1989. *Allied Health Services Avoiding Crises.* Washington, DC: National Academy Press.

———. 2000. *To Err Is Human: Building a Safer Health System.* Linda T. Kohn, Janet M. Corrigan, and Molla S. Donaldson, eds. Washington, DC: National Academy Press.

———. 2001. *Crossing the Quality Chasm: A New Health System for the 21st Century.* Washington, DC: National Academy Press.

Jordan, S. 2000. Educational input and patient outcomes: Exploring the gap. *Journal of Advanced Nursing* 31 (2):461-71.

Kaiser Family Foundation and Agency for Healthcare Research and Quality. 2000. "National Survey on Americans as Health Care Consumers: An Update on the Role of Quality Information." Online. Available at http://www.kff.org/content/2000/3093/AHRQToplines.pdf [accessed Oct. 14, 2002].

Kelly-Thomas, K. 1998. *Clincial and Nursing Staff Development.* Philadelphia, PA: Lippincott.

Long, K.A. 1994. Masters degree nursing education and health care reform: Preparing for the future. *Journal of Professional Nursing* 10 (2):71-6.

Ludmerer, K. 1999. *Time to Heal: American Medical Education from the Turn of the Century to the Era of Managed Care.* New York, NY:

Oxford University Press.

Mennin, S., and S.P. Kalishman. 1998. Issues and strategies for reform in medical education: Lessons from eight medical schools. *Academic Medicine (Supplement)* 73 (9)

Murray, E., L. Gruppen, P. Catton, R. Hays, and J.O. Woolliscroft. 2000. The accountability of clinical education: Its definition and assessment. *Medical Education* 34 (10):871-79.

National Council for State Boards of Nursing. 2001. *Report of Findings from the 2001 Employers Survey.* Chicago, IL: National Council for State Boards of Nursing.

OBrien, T., N. Freemantle, A.D. Oxman, F. Wolf, D. A. Davis, and J. Herrin. 2001. Continuing education meetings and workshops: Effects on professional practice and health care outcomes. *Cochrane Database System Review* (2): CD003030.

ONeil, E. H. and the Pew Health Professions Commission. 1998. *Recreating health professional practice for a new century - The fourth report of the PEW health professions Commission.* San Francisco, CA: Pew Health Professions Commission.

Partnership for Solutions. 2002. "Physician Concerns: Caring for People with Chronic Conditions." Online. Available at http://www.partnershipforsolutions.org/pdf_files/2002/physicianccern.pdf [accessed Oct. 8, 2002].

Platt, D., and C. Laird. 1995. CQI: Using the Hoshin planning system to design an orientation process. *Radiology Management* 17 (2):42-50.

President's Advisory Commission on Consumer Protection and Quality in the Health Care Industry. 1998. "Quality First: Better Health Care for All Americans." Online. Available at http://www.hcqualitycommission.gov/final/ [accessed Sept. 9, 2000].

Regan-Smith, M.G. 1998. "Reform without change": update, 1998. *Academic Medicine* 73 (5):505-7.

Rivo, M.L., J. Debbie M., and C.F. Lawrence. 1993. Comparing physician workforce reform recommendations. *Journal of American Medical Association* 270 (9):1083-84.

Schuster, M.A., E.A. McGlynn, and R.H. Brook. 1998. How good is the quality of health care in the United States? *Milbank Quarterly* 76 (4):517-63, 509.

Sochalski, J. 2002. Nursing shortage redux: Turning the corner on an enduring problem. *Health Affairs* 21 (5):157-64.

Weissman, J.S., E.G. Campbell, M. Gokhale, and D. Blumenthal. 2001. Residents preferences and preparation for caring for underserved populations. *Journal of Urban Health* 78 (3):535-49.

Wirthlin Worldwide. 2001 . "Pursing Perfection--Research Conducted for the Robert Wood Johnson Foundation." Online. Available at http://www.ihi.org/pursuingperfection/news/PP_Researchslides.ppt [accessed Oct. 14, 2002].

Wu, S., and A. Green. 2000. *Projection of Chronic Illness Prevalence and Cost Inflation.* California: RAND Health.

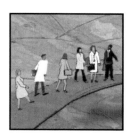

Chapter 2

Challenges Facing the Health System and Implications for Educational Reform

Major challenges face today's health care system for which health professionals have to be prepared. This chapter describes these challenges—incorporating related evidence and the views expressed by participants in the Health Professions Education Summit—and examines the resulting implications for the education of health professionals and its reform.

Current Challenges

The current quality crisis in America's heath care is well recognized. Numerous recent studies have led to the conclusion that "the burden of harm conveyed by the collective impact of all of our health care quality problems is staggering" (Chassin et al., 1998:1005). Likewise, the President's Advisory Commission on Consumer Protection and Quality in the Health Care Industry (1998: 21) note that "today, in America, there is no guarantee that any individual will receive high-quality care for any particular health problem."

The related figures are illustrative. Estimates of the number of Americans dying each year as a result of medical errors are as high as 98,000—more than those who die from motor vehicle accidents, breast cancer, or AIDS (Institute of Medicine, 2000). The American public is dissatisfied with chronic care; 72 percent of those surveyed believe it is difficult for people living with chronic conditions to obtain the necessary care from their health care providers (Harris Interactive and ARiA Marketing, 2000). Health professionals are also concerned: 57 percent of U.S. physicians surveyed said their ability to provide quality care has been reduced in the last 5 years, and 41 percent stated that they are discouraged from reporting or not encouraged to report medical errors (Blendon et al., 2001); 76 percent of nurses surveyed indicated that unsafe working conditions interfere with their ability to deliver quality care (American Nurses Association/NursingWorld.Org, 2001). A survey of over 800 physicians found that 35 percent of them reported errors in their own or a family member's care (Blendon et al., 2002).

The committee that authored the *Quality Chasm* report (Institute of Medicine, 2001), speakers at the summit, health experts, employers, and health professionals and students have all identified reasons for this disconnect between an ideal system and what actually exists. These reasons include (1) poor design of systems and processes, (2) the system's inability to respond to changing patient demographics and related requirements, (3) a failure to assimilate the rapidly growing and increasingly complex science and technology base, (4) slow adoption of information technology innovations needed to provide care, (5) little accommodation of patients' diverse demands and needs, and (6) personnel shortages and poor working conditions.

What System?

The health care system can hardly be called a system. Rather it is a dizzying array of highly decentralized sectors. Although the size of physician groups is growing, 37 percent of practicing physicians are still in solo or two-person practices (Center for Studying Health System Change, 2002). The health plan sector is turning away from structures that can facilitate integration and coordination, with the market share of health maintenance organizations (HMOs) falling and preferred provider organizations (PPOs) becoming more popular (Kaiser Family Foundation and Health Research and Educational Trust, 2002). And even though the hospital sector has been consolidating in many markets—of the 5,000 community hospitals, more than 3,500 belong to some network or system—most of these arrangements are focused on administrative rather than clinical integration (American Hospital Association, 2000; Lesser and Ginsburg, 2000). As Ken Shine, former president of the Institute of Medicine (IOM), attested at the summit:

> We operate our health care system like a cottage industry, big, big

cottages with state-of-the-art technologies to care for patients, but infrastructure which is totally inadequate, systems which don't talk to each other (Shine, 2002).

The absence of systems, or poorly designed systems, and the resulting lack of integration are apparent across sectors, as well as within individual health care organizations. Such systems can harm patients or fail to deliver what patients need. A previous IOM report makes abundantly clear that the inability to apply knowledge about human factors in systems design and the failure to incorporate well-acknowledged safety principles into health care (such as standardizing and simplifying equipment, supplies, and processes) are key contributors to the unpardonably high number of medical errors that occur (Institute of Medicine, 2000).

Mary Naylor, School of Nursing, University of Pennsylvania, a panelist at the summit, echoed this reality:

> We have both a culture and organization of care that separate our care into distinct systems—hospitals, home care, skilled nursing facilities—with little formal communication, relationships, or collaboration between and among those settings....And providers don't necessarily see that they're responsible for what happens to people as they move from one level of care to another. We don't pay a lot of attention to issues of quality assessment, particularly in those difficult hand-offs or transitions from one level of care to another (Naylor, 2002).

The *Quality Chasm* report also stresses that a redesigned system is predicated on interdisciplinary teams. In the current system, however, health professionals work together, but display little of the coordination and collaboration that would characterize an interdisciplinary team. Many factors, including differing professional and personal perspectives and values, role competition and turf issues, lack of a common language among the professions, variations in professional socialization processes, differing accreditation and licensure regulations, payment systems, and existing hierarchies, have decreased the system's ability to function, causing defined roles to predominate over meeting patients' needs. The hierarchy in which physicians dominate and the emphasis on assuming individual responsibility for decision making result in a reliance on personal accountability and a failure to solicit the contributions of others who could bring added insight and relevant information, whatever their formal credentials (Helmreich, 2000; Institute of Medicine, 2001a).

The resulting lack of continuity and coordination of care, miscommunication, redundant and wasteful processes, and excess costs have resulted in patient suffering (Institute of Medicine, 2001a; Larson, 1999). Patients and families commonly report that caregivers appear not to coordinate their work or even to know what each other are doing. Patients spend a great deal of time consulting with an endless stream of physicians, nurses, therapists, social workers, home care workers, nutritionists, pharmacists, and other specialists, who too often are ignorant of past medical histories, medications, or treatment plans and therefore work at cross purposes. When patients are moved from one setting to another—for example, from hospital to rehabilitation center to home—fragmentation of care results in overlapping or conflicting treatment that is costly and confusing and, worst of all, detrimental to the patient. In a recent survey, 85 percent of physicians surveyed stated that one or more adverse outcomes result from uncoordinated care, and more than half suggested that a lack of coordination is usually the cause of patients receiving contradictory health information from providers (Partnership for Solutions, 2002b).

Poor Accommodation of Patients' Needs

Americans are living longer, in part as a consequence of advances in medical science, technology, and health care delivery. As the population ages, there will be more patients with chronic conditions. In 2000, about 13 percent of the population (35 million Americans) were over age 65; this proportion is expected to rise to 20 percent (70 million) by 2030 (National Center for Health Statistics, 2002). An estimated 125 million Americans already have one or more chronic conditions, and more than half of these people have multiple such conditions (Wu and Green, 2000).

Moreover, although the majority of disease burden and health care resources is related to the treatment of chronic conditions, the nation's health care system is organized and oriented largely to provide acute care and is inadequate in meeting the needs of the chronically ill (Wagner et al., 2001). As William Richardson, Kellogg Foundation, noted in his remarks at the summit, "There are few clinical programs that can provide the full complement of services needed by people with heart disease, diabetes, asthma, or other common chronic conditions (Richardson, 2002).

Studies show that effective treatment of chronic conditions needs to be continuous across settings and types of providers. Clinicians need to collaborate with each other and with patients to develop joint care plans with agreed-upon goals, targets, and implementation steps. Such care should support patient self-management and encompass regular clinician follow-up, both face-to-face and through electronic means (DeBusk et al., 1994; Von Korff et al., 1997; Wagner et al., 2001; Wagner et al., 1996). Clinicians practicing in such an environment need to be effective members of an interdisciplinary team, provide care that is patient-centered, and be proficient in informatics applications.

A recent survey underscored issues faced by the chronically ill, with about three of every four respondents reporting difficulty in obtaining medical care. Specifically, 72 percent had experienced difficulty in obtaining care from a primary care physician, 79 percent from a medical specialist, and 74 percent from providers of drug therapy (Partnership for Solutions, 2002b). This same survey indicated that, as a result of the lack of coordination, the chronically ill were receiving spotty or contradictory information and facing avoidable complications. At the summit, Mary Naylor described a typical real-life example of the lack of coordination for the chronically ill:

> A 75-year old woman...had a number of chronic conditions: osteoporosis, hypertension, diabetes, and heart failure, and... was admitted to a hospital as a result of a fall...and fracture.... We followed her...from hospital admission, through one month's time, and she was the subject of about 20 major providers. That does not include the numbers of ancillary personnel and other support people involved in her care. While hospitalized, she interacted with an orthopedic surgeon and his team, a cardiologist, an endocrinologist, a primary care nurse, a physical therapist based in the hospital, and a social worker who helped facilitate her discharge to a skilled nursing facility. At that point, the hand-off was to a physician in the skilled nursing facility, a physical therapist, an occupational therapist, and a variety of other providers. Within 2 weeks' time, she was returned home to home care follow-up by the Visiting Nurse's Association, and had a nurse, occupational therapist, and physical therapist engage with her in care in the home.
>
> Her care was characterized by poor communication....Very little attention [was paid] to her preferences or the preferences of her family members in decision making about what care [she should receive] and what site she should go to, and what the plan of care should be at each of those sites. There was very poor transfer of information from one site to the other; in fact, critical pieces of her care plan were not communicated from the hospital to the nursing home, resulting in an emergency room visit within a couple of days of discharge to the skilled nursing facility. And there was no point person, no broker of care, no one there advocating for her, for her family, and coordinating this entire experience, all of which took place in a very short period of time (Naylor, 2002).

America's increasing chronic care needs also highlight the importance of health professionals being better prepared in prevention and health promotion. It has been estimated that approximately 40 percent of all deaths are caused by behavior patterns that could be modified (McGinnis et al., 2002). Prevention is also key in dealing with the nation's emerging infections, both those that occur naturally and those that are intentionally introduced. Since the events of September 11, 2001, and the anthrax attacks that followed, the once seemingly remote threat of a bioterrorist attack in the United States has now become plausible. The ability of health care professionals to apply population-based prevention strategies and activate the public health system is crucial to an effective response to such incidents. In a recent survey of health professionals, however, only a quarter of respondents said they felt prepared to respond to a bioterrorist event (Chen et al., 2002).

In addition to the need for the health system to be more responsive to those with chronic conditions and more focused on prevention, the system has not done a good job in accommodating the diverse cultural needs and varying preferences of racial and ethnic groups. A recent IOM report that reviews a large body of research concludes that racial and ethnic minorities tend to receive lower-quality care than Caucasians, even when one accounts for differences in insurance status, income, age, and severity of condition (Institute of Medicine,

2002). The IOM committee that prepared that report outlined steps needed to close this gap, including preparing health professionals to be competent in providing care that is culturally sensitive (Institute of Medicine, 2002). There is added urgency to address such inequities given that ethnic/racial minorities are predicted to comprise a majority of the U.S. population by 2050 (U.S. Census Bureau, 2002).

Inability to Assimilate the Increasingly Complex Science Base

Over the last 50 years, there has been a steady increase in funding for biomedical research that has resulted in extraordinary advances in clinical knowledge and technology. From a start of about $300 in 1887, the National Institutes of Health (NIH) has been appropriated nearly $23.4 billion for 2002 (National Institutes of Health, 2002), while investment on the part of pharmaceutical firms has risen from $13.5 billion to $24 billion between 1993 and 1999 (Pharmaceutical Research and Manufacturers of America, 2000). Likewise, research and development in the medical device industry, funded largely by private dollars, totaled $8.9 billion in 1998 (The Lewin Group, 2000). Results of all this investment include a doubling of the average number of new drugs approved each year since the 1980s (The Henry J. Kaiser Family Foundation, 2000) and exponential growth in the number of clinical trials from about 500 a year in the 1970s to more than 10,000 a year today (Chassin, 1998). There are no signs that this growth is going to abate any time soon—nor would we want that to happen.

Traditionally, it has been assumed that health professionals are able to diagnose and treat, evaluate new tests and procedures, and develop clinical practice guidelines, all using the training initially received from their academic education and ongoing practice experience. This assumption is no longer valid, with human memory becoming increasingly unreliable in keeping pace with the ever-expanding knowledge base on effective care and

its use in health care settings. For clinicians, just staying abreast of advances, let alone obtaining active training in or experience with new techniques and approaches, can be a daunting task. As David Eddy, a prominent quality expert, has said, the "complexity of modern medicine exceeds the inherent limitations of the unaided human mind" (Millenson, 1997:75). Although no practitioner needs to absorb the results of 10,000 clinical trials that span many areas of specialty, rapid expansion of knowledge is occurring even within specific areas. For example, as William Richardson noted at the summit, the number of randomized controlled trials on diabetes published over the last 30 years increased from about 5 to more than 150 per year.

Few professionals are prepared to cope with the continuously expanding knowledge and technology base, and supports to help clinicians access and apply this knowledge base to practice are not widely available. Such supports would include providing relevant information in an accessible format at the point of care. However, the literature is "replete with evidence of the failure to provide care consistent with well established guidelines for common chronic conditions" (Institute of Medicine, 2001a: 28). And the lag between the discovery of more effective forms of treatment and their incorporation into routine patient care is, on average, 17 years (Balas, 2001). Obviously, the health system needs to do better in this regard.

As William Richardson asked summit participants, "If we can't keep up now, how will we respond to the extraordinary advances that will emerge during this new century?" (Richardson, 2002). These advances include, among others, the use of genomics to diagnose and eventually treat disease; engineering discoveries such as miniaturization and robotics; and the application of advanced epidemiological knowledge, especially as it relates to bioterrorism, to large populations and databases (Institute of Medicine, 2001a).

Slow Adoption of Information Technology

Information technology is poised to bring about a significant transformation in the nation's health system, with the Internet serving as a major agent of change. The *Quality Chasm* report stresses that the automation of clinical, financial, and administrative transactions is essential to improving quality, preventing errors, enhancing consumer confidence in the health system, and improving efficiency (Institute of Medicine, 2001b). That report and others, as well as the plenary address at the summit by William Richardson, identify key areas in which a communications and information technology infrastructure could contribute greatly to enhancing the health care system (Institute of Medicine, 2001a; National Research Council, 2000). These potential contributions include enhancing clinical decision making by making real-time data available, increasing communication among providers and with patients through such approaches as remote medical consultations, collecting and aggregating clinical information and evidence into accessible information databases, facilitating patient access to reliable health information, and reducing medical errors.

Despite the range of areas in which communications and information technology could make a substantial contribution to enhancing health care access, quality, and service while reducing costs, the industry has been slow to invest in and embrace such technology. And while industries do differ in their degree of capital intensiveness, the differences in information technology investment are striking. For example, in 1996 the health care industry spent only $543 per worker on information technology, as compared with $12,666 per worker spent by securities brokers. Further, health care ranked 38th among 53 industries surveyed in terms of information technology investment (U.S. Department of Commerce, 2000).

Consequently, health care delivery has not been touched to the same degree by the revolution that has been transforming nearly every other aspect of society (Institute of Medicine, 2001a). Most clinical information is still stored in a collection of poorly organized and often illegible paper records (Staggers et al., 2001; Hagland, 2001). Few patients have e-mail access to their caregivers. Indeed, most payment to providers is based on face-to-face visits, and clinicians cannot get paid for the kinds of alternative communication that information technology offers and patients desire. Most patients do not benefit from even the simplest decision aids, such as patient reminder systems. Finally, an unacceptable number of medical errors occur because there are few information systems in place to process and check the vast amount of clinical data that flows through the system (Godin et al., 1999). In short, existing systems typically do not collect and store the right information; are not sufficiently automated or computerized; are not integrated or linked to each other; and lack the hardware, software, and data entry support necessary for retrieval and analysis of information.

One impediment to the greater use of communications and information technology is the absence of national standards for the capture, storage, communication, processing, and presentation of health information (Work Group on Computerization of Patient Records, 2000). Another is privacy and data security issues. Regulatory requirements governing e-mail use with patients, such as the Health Insurance Portability and Accountability Act, designed to help guarantee the privacy and confidentiality of patient medical records, will help somewhat in this regard. However, the *Quality Chasm* report emphasizes that in the absence of a national commitment and financial support for building a national health information infrastructure, progress in this area will be painfully slow.

Failure to Address Growing Consumerism Among Patients

There has been a growing consumerism in health care, exemplified by increases in access to health information on the Internet and other media (Calabretta, 2002; Frosch and Kaplan, 1999; Gerteis et al., 1993; Mansell et al., 2000; Mazur and Hickam, 1997). Largely as a result of the Internet, patients and their families are now better educated and informed about their health care. As a consequence, some patients want to be able to make their own decisions about diagnosis and treatment, bringing their own information and values to bear, with the expectation that, together with their health care providers, they will manage their illness or disease (Benbassat et al., 1998). In one survey, only 16 percent had sought health information via the Internet (Tu, 2003). While in another, 76 percent of respondents said they had searched the Internet for health information (Taylor, 2002). In that survey, 83 percent of respondents said they would like the results of their laboratory tests to be available online, and 69 percent expressed their desire for online charts for use in monitoring their chronic conditions over time. An annual Harris Interactive Survey spanning 1998–2002 shows a steady rise in adults who sometimes look for health information online. One survey showed that individuals span the education and income spectrum (Taylor, 2002) while another showed that higher educated individuals are more likely to search the Internet for health information (Tu, 2003).

Many patients, however, have expressed frustration with their inability to participate in decision making, to obtain the information they need, to be heard, and to participate in systems of care that are responsive to their and their families' and caregivers' needs and values (Partnership for Solutions, 2002a). Studies have demonstrated substantial shortcomings among health professionals in understanding and communicating with patients (Laine and Davidoff, 1996; Meryn, 1998; Stewart et al., 1999), as well as in their ability to provide adequate information for informed decision making (Braddock et al., 1999). An early important study revealed that in 69 percent of visits, physicians did not allow patients to complete their opening statement of symptoms and concerns, interrupting after a mean time of 18 seconds. Patients were given the opportunity

to state their full list of concerns in only 23 percent of visits (Beckman and Frankel, 1984). A later study on the same topic revealed similar results, with failure to obtain the patient's complete agenda resulting in late-arising concerns and missed opportunities to collect potentially valuable information (Marvel et al., 1999).

At the summit, Myrl Weinberg, National Health Council, attested to the problems from a patient's perspective:

> What are the complementary alternatives, treatments, over-the-counter kinds of treatments that people are taking that [are] never asked about? So often, no one ever asks. And if people are asked… they don't understand the question, and they think they're not taking any other prescription drugs and that's the end of it….Some of the studies are showing that the reason people pay billions of dollars for complementary alternative products through health food stores is because they feel a sense of shared values; that there's a holistic approach for some of these other health care providers or treatments. And they feel more comfortable there than they do any longer with individuals in the more traditional health care systems….It's not often the health care provider says, "Gee, I can't know it all, there's no way, there are other great educational sources, and here are some places you can go or Web sites that you can trust, to find out more about your condition so that we can discuss it when you're here (Weinberg, 2002)."

Workforce Shortages and Discontent

Health care has always been subject to trends in oversupply and undersupply of various health professionals, but the current shortage of nurses is different, with many experts saying it will not be resolved quickly (Buerhaus, 2000). In the year 2000, the nursing shortage was estimated at 6 percent, with 1.89 million full-time registered nurses in the workforce and demand projected at 2 million. If trends continue, the shortage is predicted to skyrocket to 29 percent by 2020 (Health Resources and Services Administration, 2002). Fully 75 percent of all current vacancies at hospitals are for nurses (American Hospital Association, 2001). Though enrollments in entry-level baccalaureate programs in nursing increased in fall 2001, ending a 6-year period of decline, the number of students in the educational pipeline is still insufficient to meet the projected demand for the million new nurses needed over the next 10 years (American Association of Colleges of Nursing, 2002). These problems are exacerbated by an increasing shortage of nursing faculty. According to the American Association of Colleges of Nursing (AACN), of more than 9,000 faculty at AACN-member nursing schools, only slightly more than 50 percent have a doctorate, and there is a large decrease in the number of nursing students with a master's degree who are pursuing academic careers (Berlin and Sechrist, 2002).

Nurses also are increasingly dissatisfied once they are on the job. A 2001 survey reveals that 40 percent of nurses working in hospitals are dissatisfied with their jobs, and 1 of 3 hospital nurses under the age of 30 is planning to leave his or her current job in the next year (Aiken et al., 2001). Sources of dissatisfaction include working conditions, such as inadequate staffing and higher use of less-skilled workers; heavy workloads; increases in overtime; a lack of sufficient support staff; and inadequacy of wages (U.S. General Accounting Office, 2001).

The nursing shortage and dissatisfaction of registered nurses with their work environments have taken a toll. An increasing number of studies have shown that patient safety issues and adverse health outcomes result, including patient deaths, as well as increased stress (physical and psychological), burnout, and frustration among health professionals (Aiken et al., 2002; Blegen et al., 1998; Buerhaus, 2000; Flood and Diers, 1998; Kovner and Gergen, 1998; Lichtig et al., 1999; Sochalski, 2002).

The shortages have resulted in fragmentation of care, with fewer opportunities for one-on-one contact between patients and health professionals.

Shortages in pharmacy are also pressing and have been characterized as "dynamic," with demand for pharmacy services increasing in recent years despite a steady growth in supply (Department of Health and Human Service, 2000; Knapp and Livesey, 2002). The shortage is attributable to a number of factors, including patients' increased use of medications; expansion of pharmacists' traditional roles to include patient education, counseling, and medication management; limited use of technology and pharmacy technicians, as well as poor work design; and greater numbers of female pharmacists, who work fewer hours than their male counterparts (Cooksey et al., 2002). There are conflicting reports on whether the shortage will be long term (Cooksey et al., 2002; Bureau of Labor Statistics. Pharmacists, 2000; Knapp, 1999).

While experts disagree about whether there is a shortage of physicians (Cooper, 2002; Cooper et al., 2002), physicians are increasingly dissatisfied with their work life. Of some 1,900 recently surveyed physicians, 27 percent anticipated leaving their practices within 2 years, with 29 percent of those being aged 34 or younger (Pathman et al., 2002). In another survey, 31 percent expressed worry that they were "burning out" as physicians (Shearer and Toedt, 2001). In Massachusetts, substantial numbers of physicians surveyed were planning to leave the state, change careers, or retire early as a result of the current practice environment (Massachusetts Medical Society Online, 2001).

While there are shortages of some health professionals, there is an increasing number of professionals in other disciplines now joining the ranks who are redefining care delivery. Nurse practitioners, certified nurse midwives, physician assistants, optometrists, podiatrists, and nurse anesthetists have all increased in number significantly in recent years (Cooper et al., 1998), though poor national data hamper accurate tabulations (Phillips et al., 2002).

Regardless, such professionals' responsibilities are increasingly overlapping with or complementing those of physicians and nurses. This situation is resulting in tremendous friction among the professions over practice control and compensation (Phillips et al., 2002), some of which gets played out in legislative battles over scope of practice.

Implications for Health Professions Education

The challenges highlighted above call for new roles and new approaches on the part of health professionals. For one thing, to care effectively for patients, the successful health professional in this century will need to master information technology, using its capabilities to manage information and access the latest evidence. Moreover, as patients arrive with better and more information from the Internet and increasingly insist that their desires, needs, and values be met, health care professionals will be called upon to modify their roles to include those of counselor, coach, and partner. Providing the high levels of coordination and collaboration needed for the chronically ill while addressing staff shortages will require that health professionals work in interdisciplinary teams, learning how to allocate responsibility effectively and provide the appropriate skill mix in a variety of settings and situations. Health professionals must also have a grasp of design and quality improvement principles so they can streamline and standardize processes for better safety and quality.

As emphasized in the *Quality Chasm* report, health professionals are working in a system that often does not support them in delivering the highest-quality care based on the latest science, let alone care that pleases patients (Institute of Medicine, 2001a). The report sets forth a framework for how the system might be transformed to close the chasm that exists between what we know to be good-quality care and what the system actually provides.

At the core of a redesigned health care system are health professionals. The effectiveness of a system in responding to patient needs depends upon a variety of factors–facilities, supplies, state of knowledge, information technology—but such inputs are meaningless without appropriately educated professionals working within and continually redesigning the system to adapt to ongoing and future challenges. Implementing the agenda set forth in the *Quality Chasm* report will necessitate fundamental changes in health professions education. Health professionals, both those in academic settings and those already in practice, must be educated differently so that they can function as effectively as possible in a reformed health care system—one focused on enhancing quality and safety. Most important, professionals will need to break down the silos that exist within the system, and seek to understand what others offer in order to do what is best for the patient. Further, health professionals must be given the tools that will empower them to make ongoing changes in the system that will continuously enhance care for patients. Although the need is pressing, major challenges face those who would reform health professions education. A number of those challenges are cited in the *Quality Chasm* report (Institute of Medicine, 2001a) and were echoed at the Health Professions Education Summit:

- A lack of funding to review curriculum and teaching methods and of the resources required to make needed changes

- Too much emphasis on research and patient care in many academic settings, with little reward for teaching

- A lack of faculty and faculty development to ensure that faculty will be available at training sites and able to teach students new competencies effectively

- No coordinated oversight across the continuum of education, and fragmented responsibilities for undergraduate and graduate education

- No integration across oversight processes, including accreditation, licensing, and certification

- The lack of an evidence base assessing the impact of changes in teaching methods or curriculum

- A shortage of visionary leaders

- Silo structures and long-standing disciplinary boundaries among and across the professions

- Unsupportive culture and norms in health professions education

- Overly crowded curricula and competing demands

- Insufficient channels for sharing information and best practices

In short, these challenges have prevented the educational system from doing a better job at meeting the requirements of the delivery system. Leaders and managers of hospitals, health plans, and health care practices cite increasing skill deficits in their workforces, including technical and computer skills, critical thinking, communication, management, delegation, supervision skills, and a systems perspective (Allied Health Workforce Innovations for the 21st Century Projects, 1999; Institute of Medicine, 2000; National Council for State Boards of Nursing, 2001). Recent graduates of educational programs cite similar skill deficits in their preparation for modern health care careers (Blumenthal et al., 2001; Cantor et al., 1993).

Conclusion

The above review of the dominant challenges facing health care suggests several key findings:

- **Poor systems design has led to errors, poor quality of care, and dissatisfaction among patients and health professionals.**

- **The needs of the chronically ill are not being adequately met. Addressing those needs requires the reform of systems of care and greater coordination and collaboration among health**

professionals, as well as more attention to prevention and the behavioral determinants of health.

- **Technological advances in information technology and an expanded evidence base gained from research on clinical practice have the potential to transform health care, but such advances have not been adequately harnessed.**

- **Patients and consumers are now increasingly informed about their health. As a result, there is a need for a new relationship of shared decision making between patients and health care providers. Providers also need to be more attentive to patient values, preferences, and cultural backgrounds.**

- **Workforce issues related to shortages and effective deployment of existing professionals need to be addressed before quality of care is further compromised.**

- **Health care employers and recent graduates cite gaps between the way health professionals are prepared and what they are called upon to do in practice, gaps that are attributable to many factors, including a lack of funding to revamp curricula and a limited focus on teaching in academic health centers.**

The *Quality Chasm* report, echoed by each of the plenary speakers at the summit, calls upon the clinical education community to provide transformational leadership in response to the challenges outlined above. At the summit, Don Berwick, Institute for Healthcare Improvement, described the purpose of the health care system—initially articulated by the President's Advisory Commission on Consumer Protection and Quality in the Health Care Industry—as continually reducing the burden of illness, injury, and disability and improving the health status and functioning of the U.S.

population. He added:

> The success of the American professional [health] education system is its ability to achieve this and nothing else. It's asking the American [health] professional education community to adopt this as 'true North' (Berwick, 2002).

Also at the summit, Ken Shine called upon health professionals to establish themselves as leaders on behalf of the American people by improving the quality of care. He added:

> Doing that is not just a self-serving activity. It's one which all of society will cherish and benefit from, and I believe it's a message which our students will respond to if they are properly motivated and have the proper insights (Shine, 2002).

These statements were intended to be a catalyst for health summit participants as they identified strategies and actions at both the institutional and environmental levels for bringing about educational reform in line with the vision for a 21st-century health system set forth in the *Quality Chasm* report. Don Berwick acknowledged the tremendous difficulties involved in bringing about change in the environment of health care and clinical education, but underscored the importance of the effort:

> You can't just say the environment won't let you do it. You just can't. It's passing the buck a step beyond what a proud set of professionals ought to be doing. We need to own it. We need to change it. We just need to change it. And if the environment is throwing us a curve ball, we just need to learn how to hit curve balls.

References

Aiken, L.H., S.P. Clarke, and D.M. Sloane. 2002. Hospital staffing, organization, and quality of care: Cross-national findings. *International Journal for Quality in Healthcare* 14 (1):5-13.

Aiken, L.H., S.P. Clarke, D.M. Sloane, J.A. Sochalski, R. Busse, H. Clarke, P. Giovannetti, J. Hunt, A.M. Rafferty, and J. Shamian. 2001. Nurses reports on hospital care in five countries. *Health Affairs* 20 (3):43-53.

Allied Health Workforce Innovations for the 21st Century Projects. 1999. "The Hidden Health Care Workforce: Recognizing, Understanding and Improving the Allied and Auxiliary Workforce." Online. Available at http://futurehealth.ucsf.edu/AHexecsum.html

American Association of Colleges of Nursing. 2002. "Enrollments Rise at U.S. Nursing Colleges and Universities Ending a Six-Year Period of Decline." Online. Available at http://www.aacn.nche.edu/Media/NewsReleases/enrl01.htm [accessed 2002].

American Hospital Association. 2000. Resource Center Fact Sheet. Fast Facts on U.S. Hospitals. *Hospital Statistics, 2000.* Chicago, IL: Health Forum - An American Hospital Association Company.

American Hospital Association. 2001. The hospital workforce shortage: immediate and future. *Trend Watch* 3 (2):1-8.

American Nurses Association/NursingWorld.Org. 2001. "On-line Health and Safety Survey: Key Findings." Online. Available at http://nursingworld.org/surveys/keyfind.pdf [accessed 2002].

Balas, E.A. 2001. Information systems can prevent errors and improve quality. *Journal of the American Medical Informatics Association* 8 (4):398-99.

Beckman, H.B., and R.M. Frankel. 1984. The effect of physician behavior on the collection of data. *Annals of Internal Medicine* 101 (5):692-6.

Benbassat, J., D. Pilpel, and M. Tidhar. 1998. Patients preferences for participation in clinical decision making: A review of published surveys. *Behavorial Medicine* 24 (2):81-88.

Berlin, L.E., and K.R. Sechrist. 2002. The shortage of doctorally prepared nursing faculty: A dire situation. *Nursing Outlook* 50 (2):50-56.

Berwick, D. 2002. "Crossing the Quality Chasm: Next Steps for Health Professions Education; Keynote Address." Online. Available at http://www.kaisernetwork.org/health_cast/hcast_index.cfm?display=detail&hc=601

[accessed Nov. 12, 2002].

Blegen, M.A., C.J. Goode, and L. Reed. 1998. Nurse Staffing and Patient Outcomes. *Nursing Research* 47 (1):43-50.

Blendon, R.J., C.M. DesRoches, M. Brodie, J.M. Benson, A.B. Rosen, E. Schneider, D.E. Altman, K. Zapert, M.J. Herrmann, and A.E. Steffenson. 2002. Views of practicing physicians and the public on medical errors. *N Engl J Med* 347 (24):1933-40.

Blendon, R.J., C. Schoen, K. Donelan, R. Osborn, C. M. DesRoches, K. Scoles, K. Davis, K. Binns, and K. Zapert. 2001. Physicians views on quality of care: A five-country comparison. *Health Affairs* 20 (3):233-43.

Blumenthal, D., M. Gokhale, E.G. Campbell, and J. S. Weissman. 2001. Preparedness for clinical practice: Reports of graduating residents at academic health centers. *Journal of the American Medical Association* 286 (9):1027-34.

Braddock, C.H.3., K.A. Edwards, N.M. Hasenberg, T.L. Laidley, and W. Levinson. 1999. Informed decision making in outpatient practice: Time to get back to basics. *Journal of American Medical Association* 282 (24):2313-20.

Buerhaus, P. 2000. A Nursing Shortage Like None Before. *Creative Nursing* 6 (2):4-8.

Bureau of Labor Statistics. Pharmacists. 2000. *Occupational Outlook Handbook*. Washington, DC: U.S. Department of Commerce.

Calabretta, N. 2002. Consumer-driven, patient-centered health care in the age of electronic information. *Journal of Medical Library Association* 90 (1):32-37.

Cantor, J.C., L.C. Baker, and R.G. Hughes. 1993. Preparedness for practice. Young physicians views of their professional education. *JAMA* 270 (9):1035-40.

Center for Studying Health System Change. 2002. "CTSonline: Physician survey results." Online. Available at http://www.hschange.com/index.cgi?file=cts1 [accessed 2002].

Chassin, M.R. 1998. Is health care ready for Six Sigma quality? *Milbank Quarterly* 76 (4):565-91, 510.

Chassin, M.R., R.W. Galvin, and the National Roundtable on Health Care Quality. 1998. The urgent need to improve health care quality. *Journal of the American Medical Association* 280 (11):1000-1005.

Chen, F.M., J. Hickner, K.S. Fink, J.M. Galliher, and H. Burstin. 2002. On the front lines: family physicians preparedness for bioterrorism. *Journal of Family Practice* 51 (9):745-50.

Cooksey, J.A., K.K. Knapp, S.M. Walton, and J.M. Cultice. 2002. Challenges to the pharmacist profession from escalating pharmaceutical demand. *Health Aff (Millwood)* 21 (5):182-88.

Cooper, R.A. 2002. There's a shortage of specialists: Is anyone listening? *Academic Medicine* 77 (8):761-6.

Cooper, R.A., T.E. Getzen, H.J. McKee, and P. Laud. 2002. Economic and demographic trends signal an impending physician shortage. *Health Affairs* 21 (1):140-54.

Cooper, R.A., T. Henderson, and C.L. Dietrich. 1998. Roles of nonphysician clinicians as autonomous providers of patient care. *Journal of the American Medical Association* 280 (9):795-802.

deBusk, R.F., N.H. Miller, H.R. Superko, C.A. Dennis, R.J. Thomas, H.T. Lew, W.E. Berger 3rd, R.S. Heller, J. Rompf, D. Gee, *et al.* 1994. A case-management system for coronary risk factor modification after acute myocardial infarction. *Annals of Internal Medicine* 120 (9):721-9.

Department of Health and Human Service. 2000. "The Pharmacist Workforce: A Study of the Supply and Demand for Pharmacist." Online. Available at ftp://ftp.hrsa.gov/bhpr/nationalcenter/pharmacy/pharmstudy.pdf [accessed 2002].

Flood, S.D., and D. Diers. 1998. Nurse staffing, patient outcome, and cost. *Nursing Management* 19 (5):34-43.

Frosch, D.L., and R.M. Kaplan. 1999. Shared decision making in clinical medicine: Past research and future directions. *American Journal of Preventive Medicine* 17 (4):285-94.

Gerteis, M., S. Edgman-Levitan, J. Daley, and T. Delbanco, editors. 1993. *Through the Patient Eyes*. Vol. San Francisco, CA: Josey-Bass.

Godin, P., R. Hubbs, B. Woods, M.M. Tsai, D.B. Nag, T.M. Rindfleish, P.P. Dev, and K.L.M.

Melmon. 1999. New paradigms for medical decision support and education: The Stanford health information network for education. *Topics in Health Information Management* 20 (2):1-14.

Harris Interactive and ARiA Marketing. 2000. "Healthcare Satisfaction Study--Final Report." Online. Available at http://www. harrisinteractive.com/news/downloads/ HarrisAriaHCSatRpt.PDF [accessed Oct., 2002].

Health Resources and Services Administration. 2002. "Projected Supply, Demand, and Shortages of Registered Nurses: 2000-2020." Online. Available at http://bhpr.hrsa.gov/ healthworkforce/rnproject/default.htm [accessed Aug. 28, 2002].

Helmreich, R.L. 2000. On error management: Lessons from aviation. *British Medical Journal* 320 (7237):781-85.

Institute of Medicine. 2000. *To Err Is Human: Building a Safer Health System.* Linda T. Kohn, Janet M. Corrigan, and Molla S. Donaldson, eds. Washington, DC: National Academy Press.

———. 2001a. *Crossing the Quality Chasm: A New Health System for the 21st Century.* Washington, DC: National Academy Press.

———. 2001b. *Improving the Quality of Long-Term Care.* GS Wunderlich and Peter O Kohler. Washington, DC: National Academy Press.

Institute of Medicine. 2002. *Unequal Treatment: Confronting Racial and Ethnic Disparities in Health Care .* Washington, DC: National Academy Press.

Kaiser Family Foundation and Health Research and Educational Trust. 2002. "2002 Employer Health Benefits Survey." Online. Available at http://www.kff.org/content/2002/20020905a/ [accessed Sept. 13, 2002].

Knapp, K.K. 1999. Charting the demand for pharmacists in the managed care era. *J Am Pharm Assoc (Wash)* 39 (4):531-6.

Knapp, K.K., and J.C. Livesey. 2002. The Aggregate Demand Index: Measuring the balance between pharmacist supply and demand, 1999-2001. *J Am Pharm Assoc (Wash)* 42 (3):391-8.

Kovner, C., and P.J. Gergen. 1998. Nurse Staffing Levels and Adverse Events Following Surgery in U.S. Hospitals. *Image: Journal of Nursing Scholarship* 30 (4):315-21.

Laine, C., and F. Davidoff. 1996. Patient-centered medicine. A professional evolution. *Journal of American Medical Association* 275 (2):152-6.

Larson, E. 1999. The impact of physician-nurse interaction on patient care. *Holistic Nursing Practice* 13 (2):38-46.

Lesser, C.S., and P.B. Ginsburg. 2000. Update on the nations health care system: 1997-1999. *Health Affairs* 19 (6):206-16.

Lichtig, L., R.A. Knauf, and D.K. Milholland. 1999. Some aspects of nursing on acute care hospital outcomes. *Journal of Nursing Administration* 29 (2):25-33.

Mansell, D., R.M. Poses, L. Kazis, and C.A. Duefield. 2000. Clinical factors that influence patients desire for participation in decisions about illness. *Archives of Medicine* 160:2991-96.

Marvel, M.K., R.M. Epstein, K. Flowers, and H.B. Beckman. 1999. Soliciting the patients agenda: Have we improved? *Journal of the American Medical Association* 281 (3):283-87.

Massachusetts Medical Society Online. 2001. "Physician Satisfaction Survey 2001." Online. Available at http://www.massmed.org/pages/ physiciansatisfaction.asp [accessed 2002].

Mazur, D.J. and D.H. Hickam. 1997. Patients preferences for risk disclosure and role in decision making for invasive medical procedures . *Journal of General Internal Medicine* 12:114-17.

McGinnis, J., P. Russo, and J. Knockman. 2002. The case for more active policy attention to health promotion. *Health Affairs* 21 (2):78-93.

Meryn, S. 1998. Improving communication skills: To carry coals to... *Medical Teacher* 20 (4):331-37.

Millenson, M. L. 1997. *Demanding Medical Excellence.* Chicago: University of Chicago Press.

National Center for Health Statistics. 2002. "Health, United States 2002, with health and aging chartbook." Online. Available at http://www. cdc.gov/nchs/data/hus/hus02cht.pdf [accessed 2002].

National Council for State Boards of Nursing. 2001. *Report of Findings from the 2001 Employers Survey.* Chicago, IL: National Council for State Boards of Nursing.

National Institutes of Health. 2002. "An Overview." Online. Available at http://www.nih.gov/about/NIHoverview.html [accessed Aug. 11, 2002].

National Research Council. 2000. *Networking Health: Prescriptions for the Internet.* Washington DC: National Academy Press.

Naylor, M. 2002. "Crossing the Quality Chasm: Next Steps for Health Professions Education; Panel Discussion." Online. Available at http://www.kaisernetwork.org/health_cast/hcast_index.cfm?display=detail&hc=601 [accessed Nov. 12, 2002].

Partnership for Solutions. 2002a. "Multiple Chronic Conditions: Complications in Care and Treatment." Online. Available at http://www.partnershipforsolutions.org/pdf_files/2002/multiplecoitions.pdf [accessed July 30, 2002a].

———. 2002b. "Physician Concerns: Caring for People with Chronic Conditions." Online. Available at http://www.partnershipforsolutions.org/pdf_files/2002/physicianccern.pdf [accessed Oct. 8, 2002b].

Pathman, D.E., T.R. Konrad, E.S. Williams, W.E. Scheckler, M. Linzer, and J. Douglas. 2002. Physician job satisfaction, dissatisfaction, and turnover. *Journal of Family Practice* 51 (7):593.

Pharmaceutical Research and Manufacturers of America. 2000. "PhRMA Annual Report, 2000-2001." Online. Available at http://www.phrma.org/publications/publications/annual2000/ [accessed Nov. 11, 2000].

Phillips, R.L. Jr, D.C. Harper, M. Wakefield, L.A. Green, and G.E. Fryer, Jr. 2002. Can nurse practitioners and physicians beat parochialism into plowshares? *Health Affairs* 21 (5):133-42.

Presidents Advisory Commission on Consumer Protection and Quality in the Health Care Industry. 1998. "Quality First: Better Health Care for All Americans." Online. Available at http://www.hcqualitycommission.gov/final/ [accessed Sept. 9, 2000].

Richardson, W. 2002. "Crossing the Quality Chasm: Next Steps for Health Professions Education; Plenary Session." Online. Available at http://

www.kaisernetwork.org/health_cast/hcast_index.cfm?display=detail&hc=601 [accessed Nov. 12, 2002].

Shearer, S., and M. Toedt. 2001. Family physicians' observations of their practice, well being, and health care in the United States. *Journal of Family Practice* 50 (9):751-6.

Shine, K. 2002. "Crossing the Quality Chasm: Next Steps for Health Professions Education; Plenary Session." Online. Available at http://www.kaisernetwork.org/health_cast/hcast_index.cfm?display=detail&hc=601 [accessed Nov. 12, 2002].

Sochalski, J. 2002. Nursing shortage redux: Turning the corner on an enduring problem. *Health Affairs* 21 (5):157-64.

Stewart, M., J.B. Brown, H. Boon, J. Galajda, L. Meredith, and M. Sangster. 1999. Evidence on patient-doctor communication. *Cancer Prevention Control* 3 (1):25-30.

Taylor, H. 2002. "The Harris Poll: Cyberchondriacs Update." Online. Available at http://www.harrisinteractive.com/harris_poll/index.asp?PID=299 [accessed 2002].

The Henry J. Kaiser Family Foundation. 2000. *Prescription Drug Trends - A Chartbook.* Menlo Park, CA: The Henry J. Kaiser Family Foundation.

The Lewin Group, I. 2000. *Outlook for Medical Technology Innovation: Will Patients Get the Care They Need. Report #1: The State of the Industry.* Washington, DC: Health Insurance Manufacturers Association.

Tu, H.T. and J.L. Hargraves. 2003. Seeking health care information: most consumers still on the sidelines. *Issue Brief Cent Stud Health Syst Change* (61):1-4.

U.S. Census Bureau. 2002 . "National Population Projections." Online. Available at http://www.census.gov/population/www/projections/natsum.html [accessed Fall, 2002].

U.S. Department of Commerce. 2000. "Falling Through the Net: Toward Digital Inclusion. A Report on American's Access to Technology Tools." Online. Available at http://www.ntia.doc.gov/ntiahome/digitaldivide/ [accessed Sept. 30, 2002].

U.S. General Accounting Office. 2001. "Nursing

Workforce: Emerging Nurse Shortages Due to Multiple Factors." Online. Available at http://www.gao.gov/new.items/d01944.pdf [accessed Fall, 2002].

Von Korff, M., J. Gruman, J. Schaefer, S.J. Curry, and E.H. Wagner. 1997. Collaborative management of chronic illness. *Annals of Internal Medicine* 127 (12):1097-102.

Wagner, E.H., B.T. Austin, C. Davis, M. Hindmarsh, J. Schaefer, and A. Bonomi. 2001. Improving chronic illness care: Translating evidence into action. *Health Affairs* 20 (6):64-78.

Wagner, E.H., B.T. Austin, and M. Von Korff. 1996. Organizing care for patients with chronic illness. [Review] [121 refs]. *Milbank Quarterly.* 74 (4):511-44.

Weinberg, M. 2002. ""Crossing the Quality Chasm: Next Steps for Health Professions Education"; Panel Discussion." Online. Available at http://www.kaisernetwork.org/health_cast/hcast_index.cfm?display=detail&hc=601 [accessed Nov. 12, 2002].

Work Group on Computerization of Patient Records. 2000. *Toward a National Health Information Infrastructure: Report of the Work Group on Computerization of Patient Records.* Washington, DC: U.S. Department of Health and Human Services.

Wu, S., and A. Green. 2000. *Projection of Chronic Illness Prevalence and Cost Inflation.* California: RAND Health.

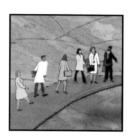

Chapter 3
The Core Competencies Needed for Health Care Professionals

Addressing the challenges outlined in Chapter 2 will require profound changes in how health systems are designed. At the heart of such systems are the skilled health care professionals without whom such a redesign could not take place. Preparing health care professionals to take on this task requires a common vision across the professions centered on a commitment to, first and foremost, meeting patients' needs as envisioned in the *Quality Chasm* report (Institute of Medicine, 2001). The committee recommends the following as an overarching vision for all programs and institutions engaged in the education of health professionals:

> *All health professionals should be educated to deliver patient-centered care as members of an interdisciplinary team, emphasizing evidence-based practice, quality improvement approaches, and informatics.*

To this end, the committee proposes a set of simple, core competencies that all health clinicians should possess, regardless of their discipline, to meet the needs of the 21st-century health care system:

- *Provide patient-centered care*—identify, respect, and care about patients' differences, values, preferences, and expressed needs; relieve pain and suffering; coordinate continuous care; listen to, clearly inform, communicate with, and educate patients; share decision making and management; and continuously advocate disease prevention, wellness, and promotion of healthy lifestyles, including a focus on population health.

- *Work in interdisciplinary teams*—cooperate, collaborate, communicate, and integrate care in teams to ensure that care is continuous and reliable.

- *Employ evidence-based practice*—integrate best research with clinical expertise and patient values for optimum care, and participate in learning and research activities to the extent feasible.

- *Apply quality improvement*—identify errors and hazards in care; understand and implement basic safety design principles, such as standardization and simplification; continually understand and measure quality of care in terms of structure, process, and outcomes in relation to patient and community needs; design and test interventions to change processes and systems of care, with the objective of improving quality.

- *Utilize informatics*—communicate, manage knowledge, mitigate error, and support decision making using information technology.

Figure 3-1 depicts the relationships among these five core competencies.

As a guide in formulating its five competencies, the committee examined core skills outlined in the *Quality Chasm* report and other core competencies formulated within and across the health professions. Following a brief review of that committee process, this chapter describes each competency in greater detail and contrasts these competencies with the corresponding current approaches in practice. Also provided is a scenario illustrating the effect on patient care when health care professionals do not apply such competencies. See Chapter 4 for more detailed discussion of the current state of practice and the implications of integrating these competencies into health professions education.

Origin of the Five Competencies

As acknowledged in the *Quality Chasm* report and in Chapter 2 of this report, there are many challenges facing health care in America. As a result, clinicians are increasingly being called upon to redesign better systems to address the health needs of the American population. The architects of the *Quality Chasm* report identify 10 important rules to guide the transition to a health system that better meets patients' needs (see Box 3-1).

The authors of the *Quality Chasm* report also foresaw that health professionals would

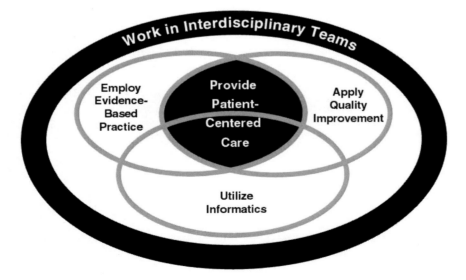

Overlap of Core Competencies for Health Professionals

Work in Interdisciplinary Teams

Employ Evidence-Based Practice

Provide Patient-Centered Care

Apply Quality Improvement

Utilize Informatics

Figure 3-1   Relationship among core competencies for health professionals.

have to perform differently to meet these rules. Thus in the chapter "Preparing the Workforce," they identified the key skills required by all health professionals to implement these new rules in the changing health care environment. The summit committee used this list of skills and the vision set forth in the *Quality Chasm* report as the foundation for its work, combining the list of skills into common groupings. The committee supplemented these groupings with a review of other seminal reform efforts that have articulated core competencies across or within the health professions. Many such efforts have emerged from the educational arena, both professional educational organizations and accreditation bodies, as well as from specialized private commissions, in response to the need to prepare the workforce adequately for the changing practice environment (ABIM Foundation, 2002; American Association of Medical Colleges, 2001; Brady et al., 2001; Center for the Advancement of Pharmaceutical Education [CAPE] Advisory Panel on Educational Outcomes, 1998; Halpern et al.,

---

Box 3-1. Ten Rules of Performance in a Redesigned Health Care System

1. Care is based on continuous healing relationships. Health professionals should provide care whenever patients need it and in many forms, not just face-to-face visits. Health professionals should be responsive at all times (24 hours a day, every day) and provide care over the Internet, by telephone, and by other means in addition to face-to-face visits.

2. Care is customized based on patient needs and values. Health professionals have the capability to respond to individual patient choices and preferences.

3. The patient is the source of control. Health professionals should be able to accommodate differences in patient preferences and encourage shared decision making.

4. Knowledge is shared, and information flows freely. Health professionals should support patients' unfettered access to their own medical information and to clinical knowledge and communicate effectively and share information with patients.

5. Decision making is evidence based. Health professionals should provide care based on the best available scientific, standardized knowledge.

6. Safety is a system property. Health professionals should ensure safety by paying greater attention to systems that help prevent and mitigate errors.

7. Transparency is necessary. Health professionals should make information available to patients and their families that allows them to make informed decisions about all aspects of care.

8. Needs are anticipated. Health professionals should be able to anticipate patient needs through planning.

9. Waste is continuously decreased. Health professionals should make efforts not to waste resources or patient time.

10. Cooperation among clinicians is a priority. Health professionals should actively collaborate and communicate to ensure an appropriate exchange of information and coordination of care.

Source: Adapted from Institute of Medicine (2001).

2001; O'Neil and the Pew Health Professions Commission, 1998).

One such major effort was undertaken by the Pew Health Professions Commission, which in 1992 articulated 17 competencies for future clinicians (O'Neil, 1992) and later expanded the list to 21 (Lenburg et al., 1999; O'Neil and the Pew Health Professions Commission, 1998). Debates centered on how to evaluate competency, focusing on the reliability, validity, and predictive ability of related measures. Nursing groups and some physicians cautioned against including only competencies that can be measured, such as those based on technical skills, as opposed to those that rely more on cognitive and critical thinking and difficult-to-assess interpersonal skills (Benner, 1982; Epstein and Hundert, 2002).

The five competencies are meant to be core and span the professions but are not intended as

an exhaustive list. The committee recognizes that there are many other competencies that health professionals should posses, such as a commitment to lifelong learning. However, the committee believes the five competencies set forth in this report are most relevant across the clinical disciplines and best advance the 10 rules envisioned in the *Quality Chasm* report. (See Table 3-1 for how the competencies address the 10 rules.)

The committee recognizes that each of the disciplines has its own contribution and unique skills to bring to patient care—this is what makes the professions unique and valuable. The five core competencies are not discipline-specific and each profession will have its own way of operationalizing such competencies in practice. However, based on patient perspectives and needs, there are certain competencies that all health professionals

Table 3-1. Rules and the Core Competencies

Rules for the 21st-Century Health System	Provide Patient-Centered Care	Employ Evidence-Based Practice	Apply Quality Improvement	Work in Inter-disciplinary Teams	Utilize Informatics
1. Care is based on continuous healing relationships.	X	X	X	X	X
2. Care is customized according to patient needs and values.	XX	X	X	X	X
3. The patient is the source of control.	X		X		X
4. Knowledge is shared, and information flows freely.	X	X	X	X	X
5. Decision making is evidence-based.	X	X	X	X	X
6. Safety is a system property.		X	X	X	X
7. Transparency is necessary.	X	X	X		X
8. Needs are anticipated.	X	X	X	X	X
9. Waste is continuously decreased.	X	X	X	X	X
10. Cooperation among clinicians is a priority.	X		X	X	X

should possess, regardless of their title or discipline.

The committee also recognizes that the definition of a professional's competency will change over time. Indeed, professionals will likely progress from novice, the stage of their initial academic preparation, to expert, the stage toward the end of their career when they have learned to do their work intuitively (Batalden et al., 2002). However, the committee is also cognizant that the fundamental competencies that define health professionals over their career are unlikely to change greatly, even though the knowledge that they must acquire, and its application, will change dramatically.

Several cautions are in order, however. First, the competencies are interrelated (see Figure 3-1), and therefore, the maximum benefit can be derived when they are applied together. Second, health professionals should apply these competencies to most clinical interactions, but they do not cover every possible clinical decision. For example, not all care is delivered by teams. Third, the following discussion of the state of application of the competencies today is not intended to be pejorative, but to capture common practices and contrast these with the committee's vision for the future.

The Five Competencies in Practice

Over the course of a lifetime, patients have numerous encounters with health care professionals. Often such encounters are effective, patients leave feeling satisfied with the care received, and their health improves. Unfortunately, this is not always the case, because health care professionals are often not supported by a system that aids them in providing optimum care. The scenario in Box 3-2, developed by the committee, is meant to illustrate some of the serious problems facing patients during an encounter with clinicians, and to show why the five core competencies outlined above are critical to improving health care. This scenario is not meant to be representative of all encounters, but is an example of a situation in which many elements have been problematic.

Box 3-2. Problematic Scenario: Mrs. Johnson

Mrs. Linda Johnson is a married first-year graduate student in her early forties with two children in high school. She made an appointment with her primary care physician, Dr. Grady, because she was always thirsty, increasingly losing weight, irritable, and fatigued.

At the end of her visit, Dr. Grady informed Mrs. Johnson that she needed to have laboratory work done to rule out the possibility of thyroid problems, anemia, or diabetes. He explained that he would call her if the results were abnormal; otherwise, she would receive a letter in the mail.

After 2 weeks of no correspondence from Dr. Grady, Mrs. Johnson called his office nurse to inquire about her test results. He returned her call the next day and apologized because her lab results had been filed in her chart instead of routed to his attention. He informed her that the test results revealed she had Type II diabetes, and she needed to make an appointment with him. Until their next visit, he advised her to watch her diet.

Twenty minutes after the scheduled time for Mrs. Johnson's next appointment, Dr. Grady entered the exam room, apologizing for the delay. During the office visit, he did not elicit additional information regarding her family history. He quickly described the long-term

(Continued on page 50)

(Continued from page 49)

complications of Type II diabetes, such as cardiovascular disease, eye disease, and kidney disease. He told Mrs. Johnson to buy a glucometer to monitor her blood sugar levels, which he explained can be controlled through dietary changes. He made an appointment for her with a dietician in 1 month. Mrs. Johnson had many questions related to how diabetes would impact her roles as a wife, mother, and graduate student, but her discussion with Dr. Grady focused on physical symptoms and he did not address her feelings or include referral to a counselor. Mrs. Johnson left the appointment feeling very frustrated and unsure of how to manage her condition.

After the visit, Dr. Grady dictated his physician notes and documented the necessary information for the diabetes registry. Because of budget constraints and workload, the updating of the diabetes registry was a month behind schedule. As a result, information from the doctor's visit and the lab values were not available for the dietician's review before she met with Mrs. Johnson.

Because of Mrs. Johnson's hectic schedule, the family diet frequently consisted of fast foods. When conducting the dietary evaluation, the dietician informed Mrs. Johnson that fast foods do not fit into a diabetic's diet. She stated that Mrs. Johnson should make it a priority to prepare well-balanced meals for her family. The dietician informed her about both good foods and bad foods that should be avoided. Her assessment was that Mrs. Johnson was overwhelmed by all the information and would not understand the concept of carbohydrates, so she did not expand on this aspect. The dietician simply encouraged her to snack on fruits and vegetables between meals. She told Mrs. Johnson that before her next visit, she wanted her to work on the changes that needed to be made in her diet. The dietician rescheduled an appointment with Mrs. Johnson in 3 months.

Mrs. Johnson purchased a glucometer from a local discount store. Not having received instructions, she was not sure that she was using the monitor properly even after calling the 1-800 number in the user manual. She brought the monitor to her local pharmacist for instructions. During this visit, the pharmacist reviewed the long-term complications of diabetes and explained the types of medications used to treat the disease, including insulin.

After visiting with the pharmacist, Mrs. Johnson read extensively about the complications of diabetes and became acutely anxious about the possibility of daily insulin injections. As a result, she drastically reduced her food intake because she thought doing so would control her blood sugar levels and prevent complications. Soon Mrs. Johnson developed sleeping difficulties and ongoing anxiety, and missed many of her graduate classes and family activities. As a result, she sought the services of a counselor at the student mental health clinic.

After her appointments with her physician, dietician, and pharmacist, Mrs. Johnson continued to have many questions about diabetes and the effect it would have on her life. Her unanswered questions included whether she should start exercising, whether she could continue to meet her responsibilities to her family, whether her diabetes would have an impact on her graduate studies, and whether she could prevent acute and long-term complications.

Mrs. Johnson's care failed on several accounts.

First, the health professionals she saw did not *provide patient-centered care*. They offered little education to help her understand her condition, such as the physical difference between Type I and Type II diabetes, the treatment process, and related complications. Mrs. Johnson and her health care providers lacked a partnering relationship in deciding how she should manage her diabetes. Her plan of care was not sufficiently individualized to account for her hectic lifestyle and issues related to being a wife, mother, and student. In addition, her providers did not address the impact the disease would have on the daily lives of her family and the family's need to understand the condition.

Second, the various health professionals did not *work as an interdisciplinary team* in the development of an individualized treatment plan for Mrs. Johnson. Her care was characterized by a lack of collaboration and communication among the doctor, laboratory personnel, the dietician, and the pharmacist. Because of the necessary interdisciplinary nature of diabetes management, a team approach is required to provide quality patient care and prevent associated long-term complications. The team must consist of the patient and all involved health care providers, for example a nurse to coordinate care, a diabetes educator for general education regarding the disease, a dietician for nutritional education, a pharmacist for medication review and education, a physician for primary care, a podiatrist for foot care, and perhaps a psychologist to address anxiety or other mental health issues.

Third, the health professionals did not *employ evidence-based practice* in Mrs. Johnson's care. The goal of diabetes education has been to promote self-management, but research has shown that knowledge alone is an insufficient predictor of an individual's ability to incorporate new self-care behaviors. Educational programs that promote effective self-care among people with Type II diabetes should be designed to foster a belief in the efficacy of self-care along with other relevant health beliefs. Strategies to this end provide the patient the opportunity to demonstrate success in the self-management of diabetes, such as mastery of the glucometer in daily usage.

Fourth, the clinic did not *apply quality improvement* methods. A diabetes registry had been implemented, but it was not being used to improve the quality of care provided to patients. The diabetes team attempted to monitor the number of patients entered into the registry, the services they received, and outcomes related to changes in their health status. Since the registry was not continuously updated, the key measures for individuals, subpopulations, and the total population were incorrectly reported. As a result, trends could not be monitored. If the diabetes registry had been continuously updated, the provider's office manager would have printed out the encounter form upon a patient's visit and clipped it to the front of the chart. This form would have provided various graphs displaying a 6-month history of care while alerting health care providers to needed tests and services. In the paper-based system that characterizes the scenario in Box 3-2, patient input depends on each health care provider's remembering to update encounter forms and office staff's having time for data entry.

Finally, health professionals did not *utilize informatics* in the clinic visited by Mrs. Johnson. Administrators in the clinic had implemented the diabetes registry, but they had not designated a specific individual to be responsible for monitoring data entry and disseminating output reports. As a result, it was impossible to know whether health care providers had failed to update the encounter forms at the time of patient visits or had delegated the paperwork to their staff, who may not have completed it correctly, if at all. When inquiries were made about updating of the encounter forms, all the health care providers stated they were positive the necessary paperwork had been completed after each visit. Yet when they received monthly reports, they believed the statistics did not correctly reflect their patient load or the number of services provided; they thought the numbers should be higher in both areas. Without an effective monitoring system in place, however, it was difficult to validate those beliefs. In sum, the paper-based system limited the health care providers' ability to search, retrieve, and manage client data from the diabetes registry.

In the following subsections, the rationale and a detailed definition for each of the five core competencies identified by the committee are presented. It should be noted that there is not in all cases a strong evidence base supporting the view that adopting a competency would result in better patient and population outcomes. Where such evidence is available, it is cited; where it is not, this lack is indicated, and the rationale for the committee's espousal of the competency is provided.

Provide Patient-Centered Care

Shifting health care needs for the American population have added a growing need for care for chronic conditions to the once predominant need for acute, episodic care. Today, 4 in 10 Americans report having a chronic condition, and by 2020, this proportion will increase to half of the nation's population (Wu and Green, 2000). Unlike those who receive acute, episodic care, patients with many coexisting conditions see a variety of health providers, in a multitude of settings, over an extended period of time. Disease-focused and clinician-centered care, which emphasizes treating a disease without attention to the needs of the patient and centers on the health professional as the sole source of control, is out of step with changing patient needs and demands. Patients are increasingly interested in customized treatment recommendations that are responsive to their preferences and beliefs and reflect an understanding of their environment, including home life, job, family relationships, cultural background, and other factors.

The health care financing system—which largely does not reimburse professionals for time spent coordinating and integrating care or providing care through alternative vehicles, such as over the Internet or via telephone— further constrains clinicians' efforts to care for patients (Institute of Medicine, 2001). Significant work done by researchers and experts in this competency area reveals specific skills needed by today's health professionals to be more responsive to patient needs (Gerteis et al., 1993; Halpern et al., 2001; Institute of Medicine, 2001; Lewin et al., 2001; Mead and Bower, 2000; O'Neil, 1992; Pew Health Professions Commission, 1995; Stewart, 2001):

- Share power and responsibility with patients and caregivers.

    - Engage in an ongoing dialogue with patients that brings about understanding, acceptance, cooperation, and identification of common goals and related care plans.

    - Guide and support those providing care to patients (e.g., family members, friends) by involving them as appropriate in decision making, supporting them as caregivers, making them welcome and comfortable in the care delivery setting, and recognizing their needs and contributions.

    - Understand and respect patients' self-management activities.

    - Provide physical comfort and emotional support.

    - Ease pain and suffering.

    - Provide timely, tailored, and expert management of symptoms.

    - Relieve fear and anxiety.

- Communicate with patients in a shared and fully open manner.

    - Allow patients to have unfettered access to the information contained in their medical records.

    - Communicate accurately in a language that patients understand. Offer trustworthy information using patients' preferred communication channels (e.g., face-to-face, e-mail, other Web-based communication technologies).

- Explore a patient's main reason for a visit, associated concerns, and need for information.

- Take into account patients' individuality, emotional needs, values, and life issues.

  - Provide care for patients in the context of the culture, health status, and health needs of the population of which each is a member.

  - Provide care that reflects the whole person.

- Implement strategies for reaching those who do not present for care on their own, including care strategies that support the broader community.

  - Accept responsibility for enrolled members of a health plan, and consider the needs of underserved members of a community who do not initiate visits or present for care.

- Enhance prevention and health promotion.

  - Apply population-based strategies to identify and reduce risk factors and to improve patients' use of and access to appropriate services and providers.

  - Define and describe populations by health status.

  - Deliver health care services intended to prevent health problems or maintain health.

  - Understand and apply principles of disease prevention and behavioral change appropriate for specific populations with which patients may identify. Understand the links among healthy lifestyles, prevention, and the cost of health care.

Multiple studies demonstrate that meeting the aim of patient-centeredness can improve health status and other outcomes desired by patients (Benbassat et al., 1998; Henbest and

Stewart, 1990; Kaplan et al., 1989; Lewin et al., 2001; Roter et al., 1995; Stewart et al., 1999). Evidence demonstrates that patients who are involved in their care decisions and management have better outcomes, lower costs, and higher functional status than those who are not so involved (Gifford et al., 1998; Superio-Cabuslay et al., 1996; Von Korff et al., 1998; Wagner et al., 2001). In a randomized controlled trial of a self-management program for chronic disease patients, participants who received the intervention showed improvement as compared with the control group in health behaviors such as frequency of exercise and improved communication with health providers, as well as improved health status and reduced hospitalization (Lorig et al., 2001). Providing patient-centered care also has been shown to lead to greater clinician satisfaction, a reduction in malpractice claims, and patient loyalty to the clinician (Meryn, 1998). Box 3-3 describes an example of care from the patient's perspective.

Providing patient-centered care is particularly important in light of the ethnic and cultural diversity that increasingly characterizes much of the United States. Although minority populations represent less than 30 percent of the national population, they constitute about 50 percent of the population in some states, such as California (Institute for the Future, 2000). A culturally diverse population poses challenges that go beyond simple language competency and include the need to understand the effects of lifestyle and cultural differences on health status and health-related behaviors; the need to adapt treatment plans and modes of delivery to different lifestyles and familial patterns; the implications of a diverse genetic endowment among the population; and the prominence of nontraditional providers, as well as family caregivers (Institute of Medicine, 2002). Box 3-4 presents an example of a system of care that is designed to respond to cultural diversity.

Researchers caution, however, that though scattered studies demonstrate positive outcomes with the provision of patient centered care, more attention needs to be paid to the methodological quality of such studies. Currently there is no

---

Box 3-3. Care From the Patient's Perspective

Planetree is a nonprofit consumer health organization dedicated to providing a model of patient-centered care through its 33 affiliate hospitals throughout the United States. The model strongly emphasizes patients having access to information regarding their illness; patient self-management and control; and healing, caring environments for patient care (Freedman, 1999).

Griffin Hospital, Derby, Connecticut, is an acute-care community hospital and a member of the Planetree Alliance. All employees at Griffin—clinical, food services, security, laboratory, pharmacy, maintenance, business office, and radiology—participate in diverse exercises designed to help them feel what it is like to be a patient, being helpless and depending on others for basic needs. At the hospital, patients document their own charts, have unrestricted visiting, and receive training for taking and charting their own medications before they are discharged home. A "care partner" program that teaches a family member to provide patient care traditionally handled only by nurses is also a feature. The physical environment is designed for healing: all patient rooms are semiprivate, with a view of the window; floors are carpeted; and art, flowers, and music figure prominently throughout the facility. Griffin's patient satisfaction rate was recently found to be 98 percent, and the facility was named one of the best companies to work for by Fortune Magazine for a third consecutive year (Griffin Hospital, 2002; Mycek, 2001).

---

gold-standard measure for patient-centeredness. The absence of valid, reliable, and appropriate tools to assess the effects of interventions to promote patient-centered care has been a large obstacle in performing such assessments uniformly (Mead and Bower, 2000). Another obstacle has been associated with the definition of terms related to this competency. Though a widely used phrase, *patient-centered care* has little shared meaning within and across the health professions. In their systematic review, Lewin and colleagues (2001) note that more work needs to be done on defining common language and terms related to patient-centered care that can be operationalized in effectiveness studies.

Work in Interdisciplinary Teams

An interdisciplinary team is composed of members from different professions and occupations with varied and specialized knowledge, skills, and methods. The team members integrate their observations, bodies of expertise, and spheres of decision making to coordinate, collaborate, and communicate with one another in order to optimize care for a patient or group of patients. It should be noted that, although patients and their caregivers are increasingly performing tasks once performed strictly by health professionals (Hart, 1995; Lorig et al., 1999; Von Korff et al., 1997) and so could be considered part of the larger health care team when they so desire, this report focuses on the educational needs of trained health professionals. Thus this competency refers to the various disciplines working together to address the needs of patients. Interdisciplinary teams are critical in dealing with the increasing complexity of care, coordinating and responding to multiple patient needs, keeping pace with the demands of new technology, responding to the demands of payors, and delivering care across settings (Bluml et al., 1999; Hall and Weaver, 2001; Institute of Medicine, 2001). Teams tend to reduce the utilization of redundant or duplicate services, and they also tend to develop more creative solutions to complex problems because of their members' diverse academic backgrounds and experience. Patients needing chronic care, critical acute care, geriatric care,

---

Box 3-4. Responding to the Diversity of the U.S. Population

In response to the rapidly changing demographic profile in the United States and rising health care costs, **Kaiser Permanente** created the **Institute for Culturally Competent Care**. The institute is devoted to creating a system of care that ensures members' cultural needs are considered and respected at every point of contact between the member and the organization. The institute facilitates operation of the Centers of Excellence in Culturally Competent Care, regional centers that successfully integrate cultural competence into their local health care delivery system.

The centers focus on two or three health issues that significantly affect a population highly represented among the local membership. The centers then develop culturally relevant care management programs designed to positively affect health outcomes of the given population. Each has a different mission and focus: African American Populations (Los Angeles), Latino Populations (Colorado), Linguistic and Cultural Services (San Francisco), Women's Health, Members with Disabilities, and Eastern European Populations.

The San Francisco center has established a department of multicultural services that provides on-site interpreters for patients in all languages, with internal staffing capability in 14 different languages and dialects. A translation unit ensures that written materials and signs are translated into the necessary languages. A cultural diversity advisory board has also been established for oversight and consultation. In addition, modules of culturally targeted health care delivery have been developed that include a multilingual Chinese module and a bilingual Spanish module, which incorporate specific cultural and linguistic capacity to care for these populations. Interdisciplinary teams, including diabetes nurses, case managers, and health educators, are emphasized.

Source: Goldsmith (2000).

---

and care at the end of life require smooth team functioning because of the complexity of their needs. Different means and settings for delivering care, such as managed care, community-based care, rehabilitation centers, and critical pathway systems, are gaining momentum and require interdisciplinary teams to provide the necessary coordination (Amsterdam et al., 1980; McDonough and Doucette, 2001; Weingart, 1996). Most but not all care should be delivered by teams, either formally or informally organized.

Interdisciplinary teams have been shown to enhance quality and lower costs in some studies (Baldwin, 1996; Burl et al., 1998; Curley et al., 1998; McDonough and Doucette, 2001; Shortell, 1994; Wagner et al., 2001). The identification or addition of team members to achieve greater concordance with complex treatment protocols on the part of both providers and patients has improved outcomes for several chronic conditions (Wagner, 2000). Studies have also demonstrated a relationship between better interaction among team members in intensive care units and decreased risk-adjusted length of stay (Shortell, 1994). Still other studies have demonstrated some impact of effective team care on patient safety and reduction of medical errors (Silver and Antonow, 2000; Weeks et al., 2001). However, more research is needed to fully explore the effect of teams on patient outcomes and cost, as well as the effectiveness of teams in ambulatory settings (Cooper and Fishman, 2003). Summit participants suggested making systematic evaluation a part of all interdisciplinary team activity as an important first step. The committee decided to focus one of its recommendations on further developing the evidence base for this and other core competencies.

Evidence is lacking on how best to distribute patient care functions within a collaborative team and how to improve clinicians' willingness or ability to collaborate (Lewin et al., 2001), as well as on the role of accrediting organizations in fostering interdisciplinary teams (Hall and Weaver, 2001). A great deal has been learned, however, about how to break down hierarchies and develop trust, and about the need for preplanning of roles. Experience has shown that being an effective team member requires health professionals to (Hall and Weaver, 2001; Halpern et al., 2001; Helmreich, 2000; Reese and Sontag, 2001):

- Learn about other team members' expertise, background, knowledge, and values.

- Learn individual roles and processes required to work collaboratively.

- Demonstrate basic group skills, including communication, negotiation, delegation, time management, and assessment of group dynamics.

- Ensure that accurate and timely information reaches those who need it at the appropriate time.

- Customize care and manage smooth transitions across settings and over time, even when the team members are in entirely different physical locations.

- Coordinate and integrate care processes to ensure excellence, continuity, and reliability of the care provided.

- Resolve conflicts with other members of the team.

- Communicate with other members of the team in a shared language, even when the members are in entirely different physical locations.

In the future health care system, health professionals will have to understand the advantage of high levels of cooperation, coordination, and standardization to guarantee excellence, continuity, safety, and reliability. In short, they will have to think of themselves as a team working in and contributing to a larger system. As Don Berwick, Institute for Healthcare Improvement, said at the summit,

> System-mindedness means cooperation. It means skills such as conflict resolution. It means asking yourself...not what are the parts of me, not what do I do, but what am I part of?

Employ Evidence-Based Practice

Using the ever-expanding evidence base, health professionals can consistently promote best practices and avoid the underuse, misuse, and overuse of care (Chassin, 1998). The committee believes it is critical for interdisciplinary health teams and each of the disciplines to be able to tap this evidence base effectively at the point of patient care, determining whether an intervention, such as a preventive service, diagnostic test, or therapy, can be expected to produce better outcomes than alternatives—including the alternative of doing nothing.

The notion of evidence-based practice refers to the integration of best research evidence, clinical expertise, and patient values in making decisions about the care of individual patients (Institute of Medicine, 2001; Straus and Sackett, 1998). *Best research evidence* includes evidence that can be quantified, such as that from randomized controlled trials, laboratory experiments, clinical trials, epidemiological research, and outcomes research; evidence based on qualitative research; and evidence derived from the practice knowledge of experts, including inductive reasoning (Guyatt et al., 2000; Higgs et al., 2001). *Clinical expertise* is derived from the knowledge and experience developed over time from practice, including inductive reasoning. *Patient values and circumstances* are the unique preferences, concerns, expectations, financial resources, and social supports that are brought by each patient to a clinical encounter. This definition of evidence is inclusive—it does not mean that all decisions must be based on the results of randomized controlled trials, as such results are not always available, nor does it discount clinician experience or the integration of information about a patient's special circumstances. Rather, all such sources of knowledge may be relevant and valuable in deciding how to apply evidence. Box 3-5 presents an example of how clinicians can work in teams to apply the evidence base thus defined.

Considerable progress has been made on identifying and disseminating best research findings about effective clinical practice. Such efforts include journals that summarize primary research, the Agency for Healthcare Research and Quality's development of a national clearinghouse for clinical guidelines and launch of evidence-based practice centers to produce and disseminate evidence reports and technology assessments, the National Institutes of Health's Consensus Development Program (National Institutes of Health, 2002), and the development of secondary databases of relevant research (Jadad and Haynes, 1998; Walshe and Rundall, 2001).

The committee believes that to employ evidence in practice, health care professionals should be able to (Davidoff, 1999; Grad et al., 2001; Rosswurm and Larrabee, 1999):

- Know where and how to find the best possible sources of evidence.

Box 3-5. Working in Teams to Apply the Evidence Base

HealthEast, an integrated care delivery system including acute care, chronic care, senior services, community-based services, ambulatory/outpatient services, physician clinics, and wellness services in St. Paul, Minnesota, embarked on establishing a single organized, systemwide approach to care management. First, a series of tools was developed—pathways, standing orders, decision algorithms, and patient education materials—to guide care. Then, interdisciplinary care management teams, including nursing, social work services, and quality management, were formed to provide care coordination and discharge planning, including keeping patients on the pathway during an episode of care.

This effort also included "collaborative practice committees"—multidisciplinary oversight groups, led by various disciplines, for the improvement of care within clinical populations. Educational development of these teams was accomplished through formal introductory courses, which included background on care management, the impact of the managed care marketplace, performance improvement tools and techniques, and the collaborative practice model. Using existing clinical and financial databases and additional chart review, the groups sought to understand the current process of care within the company.

The results of this process were compared with information from the literature and with benchmarks from other organizations when possible. The collaboratives then established some broad goals for improvement, such as improved survival rates or reduced costs of care for their clinical populations, whose conditions ranged from myocardial infarction to hip fracture to asthma. The use of this model was instrumental in achieving important improvements in financial and clinical performance, including significant reductions in length of stay for certain populations.

Source: Green (1998).

- Formulate clear clinical questions.

- Search for the relevant answers to those questions from the best possible sources of evidence, including those that evaluate or appraise the evidence for its validity and usefulness with respect to a particular patient or population.

- Determine when and how to integrate these new findings into practice.

While there is evidence that the dissemination of research on effectiveness has improved patient outcomes in discrete venues, such as treatment of lower-back pain, acute myocardial infarction, and other conditions (Goldberg et al., 2001; Mehta et al., 2002), the extent to which this approach has had an effect on overall clinical practice is unclear (Jadad and Haynes, 1998; Walshe and Rundall, 2001). A large barrier is that, although the evidence base for medicine is robust and continually expanding, the evidence bases for the other professions are lacking. Nursing and allied health interventions are not captured in medical records, which provide underlying data for research studies that make up the evidence base. For example, problems of importance to nursing practice, such as patient pain, dehydration, skin breakdown, lifestyle change, knowledge deficiencies, noncompliance with therapies, and anxiety management, are largely not captured in research, clinical, and administrative data systems and so cannot be retrieved for use as evidence in practice (Lang, 1999). Another obstacle is that nursing and allied health interventions often are not evaluated using rigorous quantitative research designs, but are described in descriptive or qualitative studies (Department of Health and Human Services, 1998; Evers, 2001; Mazurek, 2002).

Nursing and allied health leaders advocate standardizing evidence in their fields and combining it with other bodies of evidence to achieve the best possible outcomes for patients and strengthening the evidence base to include more randomized studies (Denehy, 1998; Department of Health and Human Services, 1998; Lang, 1999; Zielstorff, 1998). Summit

participants suggested that focusing on common core bodies of evidence and developing a common language and consistent terminology across the professions are also key to employing evidence-based practice in health care.

Significant barriers to employing evidence-based practice include difficulty in getting research findings to practitioners in a useful format at the point of care, time constraints on the part of busy health professionals, professional ideologies that emphasize practical rather than intellectual knowledge, the notion that evidence-based practice represents a cookbook approach to care, and practice environments that do not encourage information seeking (DiCenso et al., 1998; Haynes, 2002). In response, some have proposed a greater role for specially trained clinical librarians to assist health professionals in framing clinical questions and identifying the relevant literature (Davidoff and Florance, 2000).

Many efforts are also under way to make it easier for clinicians and patients to access and interpret findings reported in the literature and apply them to practice. These include a sizable number of online databases devoted to reviews of the evidence base. Examples include the American College of Physicians (2002) Journal Club, the Cochrane Collaboration's (2001) regularly maintained reviews of evidence, the Database of Abstracts of Reviews of Effectiveness (NHS Centre for Review and Dissemination, 2002), and MEDLINE at the National Library of Medicine (2002)—the largest general biomedical research literature database. There are also various Web sites that organize information around particular health needs, such as the American Cancer Society's (2002) site; numerous journals that summarize primary research, such as *Evidence-based Medicine* and *Evidence-based Nursing*; and the Agency for Healthcare Research and Quality's (2002) evidence reviews. In addition, continuing advances in informatics, such as computerized decision support systems that remind clinicians to provide care according to the latest available evidence, are a promising development, although a meta-analysis by Hunt and colleagues (1998) suggests that the effects of such systems on patient outcomes have been insufficiently studied (Walshe and Rundall, 2001).

Apply Quality Improvement

The Institute of Medicine (IOM) has defined quality as the "degree to which health services for individuals and populations increase the likelihood of desired health outcomes and are consistent with current professional knowledge" (Institute of Medicine, 1990:4). As noted previously, two recent IOM reports—*To Err Is Human: Building a Safer Health System* (Institute of Medicine, 2000) and *Crossing the Quality Chasm: A New Health System for the 21st Century* (Institute of Medicine, 2001)—document abundant evidence of serious and extensive quality problems throughout the U.S. health care system. Poorly designed care processes or systems have led to unnecessary duplication of services, long waiting times and delays, and compromised patient safety, resulting in avoidable errors and harm to patients (Schuster et al., 1998).

In addition to an unacceptable number of errors, the health care system is plagued by waste and inefficiency. Waste involves the use of resources without benefit to patients: extra and useless tests; multiple entries of such things as physicians' prescriptions and laboratory orders; classifications that add complexity without adding value, such as types of appointments and job classifications; and multiple layers of control, such as approvals. Inefficiency is apparent in the long waits patients must endure for both services and test results. Such waiting can result in a delay in diagnosis or treatment that leads to preventable complications (Institute of Medicine, 2001).

Health care organizations are increasingly adopting methods and techniques that originated in various industrial movements, such as total quality management and continuous quality improvement, to minimize waste, decrease errors, increase efficiency, and ultimately improve quality of care. Most commonly

termed *quality improvement* in health care, these approaches require that health professionals be clear about what they are trying to accomplish, what changes they can make that will result in an improvement, and how they will know that the improvement has occurred (Berwick, 1996). More specifically, health care professionals need to be educated to do the following (Berwick et al., 1992; Donabedian, 1980; Halpern et al., 2001; Institute of Medicine, 2001; Schuster et al., 1998):

- Continually understand and measure quality of care in terms of *structure*, or the inputs into the system, such as patients, staff, and environments; *process*, or the interactions between clinicians and patients; and *outcomes*, or evidence about changes in patients' health status in relation to patient and community needs.

- Assess current practices and compare them with relevant better practices elsewhere as a means of identifying opportunities for improvement.

- Design and test interventions to change the process of care, with the objective of improving quality.

- Identify errors and hazards in care; understand and implement basic safety design principles, such as standardization and simplification and human factors training.

- Both act as an effective member of an interdisciplinary team and improve the quality of one's own performance through self-assessment and personal change.

A growing body of studies indicates that applying quality improvement methods and principles mitigates errors, waste, inefficiency, and delay (Holman et al., 2001; Kiefe et al., 2001; O'Connor et al., 1996). One study found that implementation of a quality improvement program was associated with a high level of adherence to quality-of-care indicators for acute mycordial infarction (Mehta et al., 2000). Using quality improvement methods, researchers were able to improve medication management for depression (Unutzer et al., 2001). And physicians and other health professionals involved in cardiac surgery in northern New England used continuous improvement techniques to reduce their in-hospital mortality rate after coronary artery bypass graft surgery; after 2 years, a 24 percent reduction in the in-hospital mortality rate was achieved (O'Connor et al., 1996). Box 3-6 presents an example of how interdisciplinary teams can apply quality improvement strategies to reduce errors.

Quality improvement emerged from the industrial sector as an effective package of theory and practical tools for reducing errors in the production process. As applied to health care, it has been praised by some, but has spread slowly. One notable constraint has been the lack of a supporting information infrastructure. Another has been an absence of leadership and support and a lack of enthusiasm from and often skepticism among health care providers regarding the effectiveness of the approach (Blumenthal and Epstein, 1996; Brennan, 1998; Ferlie and Shortell, 2001). Such skepticism is understandable, given that the evidence for the effectiveness of the approach is largely anecdotal (Blumenthal and Kilo, 1998), and the rigor of much of the evidence available is questionable (Shortell et al., 1998).

Regardless of the barriers outlined above, the committee believes that the question is not whether health professionals should apply quality improvement approaches, but how they can implement such approaches more successfully within health care. One review of the studies to date suggests that quality improvement approaches should be better adapted to the realities of health care and be more related to the needs of clinicians and to patient-related problems (Grol, 2001). Summit participants advocated that the health care system build on the experience of groups in other industries that have been able to demonstrate gains in quality through the use of quality improvement methods.

Utilize Informatics

Health care informatics is more than information technology; it is the development and application of information technology systems to problems in health care, research, and education (Masys et al., 2000). Informatics

---

Box 3-6. Working in Teams to Reduce Errors

Luther Midelfort Hospital in Eau Claire, Wisconsin, is a 300-bed facility, part of the Mayo Health System. An interdisciplinary team of a nurse, a physician, and a pharmacist was formed to examine medical errors in the facility. Data showed that 56 percent of the hospital's medication errors occurred during admission, in hospital transfers, and at discharge. Armed with this information, the team began applying quality improvement methods to address medication errors occurring during these three interfaces of care. They discovered variations in the use of Coumadin, a blood thinner, that resulted in patient bleeding and strokes.

The team then created nurse-run protocols and reduced the adverse events associated with the drug from 25 to 10 percent, while also reducing the number of laboratory tests by 30 percent. Another improvement was the creation of a standard scale for insulin dosage. That scale is now being used for all diabetics admitted to the hospital, leading to a 50 percent decline in insulin medication errors. As a result of such quality improvement efforts, a nonpunitive culture of error prevention is in place hospitalwide, and reports of errors from nurses and technicians are encouraged.

Sources: Rebillot (2000); Luciano (2000).

has made many contributions to the health care environment in recent years: applications of information technology to administrative and financial transactions, such as billing and ordering; a virtual explosion of health-related information available to consumers via the Internet; and gains in making syntheses of evidence, practice guidelines, and health services research more accessible to health professionals, researchers, and patients. Informatics has begun to be applied more directly to the clinical realm as well through such applications as reminder and decision support systems, order entry systems, telemedicine, teleradiology, online prescribing, and e-mail. Box 3-7 describes the efforts of one government program to improve quality through the use of informatics. The committee believes, and past research has shown, that through the

utilization of such tools, health professionals will be able to perform four key tasks—reduce errors, manage knowledge and information, make decisions, and communicate—more effectively than has been the case in the past.

Reduce Errors

Information system applications have been shown to enhance patient safety by standardizing and automating certain decisions and by flagging errors, such as adverse drug interactions, before they are allowed to occur. Likewise, computerized medical records, with their elimination of handwritten data, are integral to error reduction. Computerized prescriber order entry systems can eliminate errors caused by misreading or misinterpreting handwritten instructions. They also can

---

Box 3-7. Quality Improvement and Informatics Leading to Better Patient Outcomes

The Veterans Health Administration (VHA) operates the largest health care system in the nation, providing care at more than 1,200 sites, including 172 medical centers and more than 600 outpatient clinics. The VHA has set the benchmark in patient safety and improved patient outcomes through a variety of quality improvement and informatics interventions in the last decade.

At the heart of the VHA's informatics efforts is the Computerized Patient Record System (CPRS), which integrates all clinical data needed to support clinical decision making. Among its many functions, the system reminds health care workers to provide routine services, such as immunizations and cancer screening, at the point of care. All VHA facilities also use electronic entry of prescriptions to eliminate mistakes from illegible handwriting. Additionally, the VHA is the first health care system in the nation to use a bar-code system for medication, similar to the computerized codes in stores, which has cut medical errors by two-thirds. In addition to provider-oriented informatics applications, the VHA has established My Healthy Vet, which provides veterans an online connection to their medical records.

In its effort to improve quality, the VHA created the National Surgical Quality Improvement Program in 1991 to provide systematic insight into surgical care and to improve surgical outcomes. During the last 5 years, this program has led to a 10 percent reduction in mortality and a 30 percent reduction in postoperative complications. In 1995, the VHA created a performance measurement system that monitors adherence to clinical practice guidelines and measures clinical outcomes. The VHA also is requiring health care workers to attend 40 hours of instruction on quality improvement as part of their continuing education.

Source: Khuri et al. (2002).

---

intercept orders that might result in adverse drug reactions or that deviate from standard protocols. One study found that the use of a physician order entry system resulted in a 55 percent reduction in medical errors and a 17 percent decrease in the preventable adverse drug event rate (Bates et al., 1998); 80 percent of medication errors unrelated to missed dosage were also found to be eliminated by such systems (Bates et al., 1999). Computer-generated reminders have been shown to be effective in reducing errors of omission as well (Overhage et al., 1997). E-mail communication, electronic medical records, and computer-aided decision support systems also offer the potential to improve care across clinicians and settings, thus reducing the chances of errors resulting from poor coordination (Blumenthal, 1997). One example of the use of online patient registries is described in Box 3-8.

Manage Knowledge and Information

Online databases can make it possible for health professionals to access the knowledge base and literature sources needed to conduct evidence-based practice (Gambrill, 1999). Onsite computerized databases or disease registries can enable the meticulous collection of personal health information throughout a patient's life, which health professionals can access to manage the many forms of chronic illness that require frequent monitoring and ongoing patient support (Bodenheimer et al., 2002). Electronic medical records, which can be held physically or digitally in a variety of locations, can make the latest information available for patients and health professionals (Institute of Medicine, 1997; Masys et al., 2002). Many electronic medical records feature computer prompting that asks for missing information and therefore enables more complete documentation (Raymond and Dold, 2002).

Make Decisions

Computerized decision support systems serve as reminders to help primary care teams comply with evidence-based practice guidelines or as sources of feedback to providers to show how they are performing on various care

---

Box 3-8. Use of Online Registries

Group Health Cooperative of Puget Sound (GHC) has developed online registries for diabetes, heart care, depression, breast cancer, and pediatric immunizations. The registries provide member-level clinical data for those with the targeted conditions, including dates of visits for recommended preventive services, results of laboratory tests, and prescriptions, as well as other key information, such as risk factors (e.g., smoking) and patient contact information. They also show red flags when the results of a laboratory test are abnormal or recommended visit schedules have not been met (e.g., a diabetic patient is overdue for an eye exam). Physicians can enter and correct patient information in the registry to monitor progress toward improvement goals for these populations.

In one district, office nurses reportedly use the registries to generate timed, proactive letters to patients who are due to receive laboratory tests. Nurses most often take responsibility for keeping the registries accurate and actively using them in outreach to members who need care. GHC's intranet contains patient education brochures on at least 20 clinical topics, the plan's practice guidelines and supporting information at optional levels of detail drawn from the evidence, and a database of pharmacy information on plan members. A year after it was made available, 80 percent of physicians had logged on to the diabetes registry.

Sources: Felt-Lisk and Kleinman (2000); McCulloch et al. (1998); Wagner et al. (2001).

measures (Bodenheimer et al., 2002). Such systems have been effective in encouraging physician compliance with recommended guidelines that support improved drug prescribing, dosing, and administration; treatment; and prevention and monitoring (Bates et al., 1999; Cooley et al., 1999; Evans et al., 1998; Hunt et al., 1998; Lobach and Hammond, 1997). In a meta-analysis of 33 studies on the effect of prompting clinicians, 25 of which used computer-generated reminders, the technique was found to enhance performance significantly for all 16 preventive care procedures studied (Balas, 2001).

Communicate

By communicating via e-mail and accessing their electronic medical records and hospital information systems via the Internet, patients can share and exchange with health providers information about their general health, symptoms, and concerns. Likewise, clinicians can use their knowledge and skills to respond with pertinent medical information, and in many cases reassurance (Brotherton et al., 2001; Jadad and Haynes, 1998; MacDonald et al., 2001). Using e-mail, health providers can also send appointment reminder messages, discuss a prescription renewal, and notify patients of test results. The creation of communities of patients and clinicians with shared interests is also enabled through the Internet, facilitating the self-management needed for better disease management (Cain et al., 2000; Houston and Ehrenberger, 2001).

There is ongoing debate among the health professions as to whether informatics is discipline-specific, requiring distinct core curricula, training programs, and professional identities (Masys et al., 2000). Nonetheless, the committee agrees that all health professionals need the following general informatics competencies, regardless of their discipline (Bader and Braude, 1998; Mallow and Gilje, 1999; Masys, 1998; Saba, 2001; Saranto and Leino-Kilpi, 1997; Sinclair and Gardner, 1999):

- Employ word processing, presentation, and data analysis software.

- Search, retrieve, manage, and make decisions using electronic data from internal information databases and external online databases and the Internet.

- Communicate using e-mail, instant messaging, listservs, and file transfers.

- Understand security protections such as access control, data security, and data encryption, and directly address ethical and legal issues related to the use of information technology in practice.

- Enhance education and access to reliable health information for patients.

In addition to improving the quality of health care, information technology has significant potential for use in measuring the level of performance of health care providers. Specifically, information technology can facilitate the collection of process and outcome data that can be used to assess of the competency of health care professionals (Blendon et al., 2002).

The committee acknowledges that certain legal and regulatory issues need to be addressed before widespread utilization of informatics becomes a reality. The regulatory requirements governing e-mail use with patients, such as the Health Insurance Portability and Accountability Act (Centers for Medicaid and Medicare Services, 2002), are designed to help guarantee the privacy and confidentiality of patient medical records. Achieving compliance with such standards, particularly for health care providers, means that future and currently practicing health professionals must be educated and trained in technologies for protecting access to provider–patient communications. Evolving issues related to the use of informatics by health care professionals include the need for standards for data so that they can be shared across settings, decisions about who should have access to patient-based information, documentation of provider–patient communications in patient records, and medical practice liability concerns (National Committee on Vital and Health Statistics, 2000).

Box 3-9. Applying All Competencies for Quality Care

Wagner and colleagues (Wagner, 1998; Wagner et al., 1996) have developed a Chronic Care Model that guides health care providers in efficiently managing the care of patients with chronic illness. Using the model, health professionals collaborate and involve patients in decisions, with patients directly controlling their diet, exercise, and medication. The model also emphasizes interdisciplinary teams—physicians treat patients with acute problems, while other professionals support patient self-management, arrange for routine periodic tasks, and ensure appropriate follow-up. The teams employ evidence-based practice guidelines supported by informatics. Computerized reminder systems help teams comply with practice guidelines; feedback systems show how each patient is performing on chronic illness measures; and computerized disease registry systems help teams plan and improve individual patient and population-based care. More than 300 diverse health care systems are introducing elements of the model in the context of quality improvement collaboratives for asthma, congestive heart failure, depression, diabetes, and prevention of frailty in the elderly.[1]

Clinica Campesina, a community health center providing care to a largely uninsured Hispanic population around Denver, Colorado, joined the diabetes collaborative in 1998. The interdisciplinary team established a patient registry, enabling them to learn which of their patients had poorly controlled diabetes or difficulty coming to the clinic. Using this information, the team is able to regularly provide outreach to patients, including through diabetes fairs in the community. Employing evidence-based guidelines, the team developed a flow sheet with simple algorithms of care for providers. The team encourages patients to manage their illness through diabetes education and collaborative setting of diabetes treatment goals during each clinic visit.

Premier Health Partners joined the collaborative in 1998. Premier is a complex integrated health system with two hospitals, 100 private practices, a long-term care facility, and a home health agency in Dayton, Ohio. Developing and employing evidence-based practice, diabetes guidelines, academic detailing, and a toolkit of printed materials that incorporates the guidelines into the day-to-day care of diabetic patients, providers are able to support patient self-management, including individual and group classes and flowcharts on which patients record their own laboratory test results. Interdisciplinary teams of physicians and nurses work to monitor the diabetes flow sheets. Computerized medical record reviews in each primary care practice generate physician-specific data on diabetes measures and are then circulated to providers. The information system will soon be generating physician and patient reminders.

Outcomes for both settings, described above, have shown substantial increases in preventive measures for patients, such as eye and foot exams, better glycemic control, lower HgA1C, and substantial increases in the percentage of diabetic patients with at least two hemoglobin tests within a year (Bodenheimer et al., 2002; Institute for Healthcare Improvement and National Coalition on Health Care, 2002).

---

[1] The Health Disparities Collaborative is a joint effort by the Bureau of Primary Health Care, The Robert Wood Johnson Foundation's project Improving Chronic Illness Care (Robert Wood Johnson Foundation, 2002), the Institute for Healthcare Improvement, and the National Association of Community Health Centers to improve health outcomes for medically underserved people with chronic diseases.

A Vision of the Prepared Health Care Professional

The core competencies described in this chapter can lead to fundamentally better care. Having begun in this chapter with a scenario that depicts a patient encountering significant deficits and gaps in care (Box 3-2), we conclude with a scenario developed by the committee that depicts care as it could be if health care providers exhibited the five competencies (Box 3-10).

Mrs. Johnson's health care needs were met in several ways.

First, health professionals provided *patient-centered care* as they shared information on the decision-making process and the management of diabetes with the patient. It was evident that Mrs. Johnson valued her education and family. In the interdisciplinary team meeting, she voiced her frustration regarding the amount of time it was taking her to learn how to self-

manage her diabetes while attempting to meet her responsibilities as wife, mother, and graduate student. She was fearful that she would have to quite graduate school. The interdisciplinary team members reviewed Mrs. Johnson's short-term self-management goals with her and emphasized her successes. In addition, they discussed options that would allow her to meet her varied responsibilities. By the end of the interdisciplinary team meeting, Mrs. Johnson felt confident that she was making progress in the self-management of her condition. In addition, she and her husband decided that instead of quitting graduate school, she should decrease her course load to one class per semester until she felt comfortable with juggling the self-management of her diabetes and her other responsibilities.

Second, the health professionals *worked in an interdisciplinary team* in approaching Mrs. Johnson's care. She was referred to a number of health care providers who offered education

---

Box 3-10. Future Scenario: Mrs. Johnson

Mrs. Linda Johnson is a married first-year graduate student in her early forties with two children in high school. She made an appointment with her primary care physician, Dr. Grady, because she was always thirsty, losing weight, irritable, and extremely fatigued.

After having her history taken and undergoing a physical exam, as well as thorough laboratory testing, Mrs. Johnson was diagnosed with Type II diabetes. Dr. Grady elicited a family history of diabetes and learned Mrs. Johnson had an uncle with Type I diabetes who suffered severe complications from this chronic disease. Dr. Grady explained the physiology of diabetes, the differences between Type I and Type II, acute and chronic complications, necessary laboratory tests, and normal values. He advised Mrs. Johnson to purchase a glucometer for daily blood sugar monitoring.

Dr. Grady explained that the treatment of her diabetes would require a partnership between Mrs. Johnson and an interdisciplinary team of health care providers. He stated that the ultimate goal of the team would be to help her manage her diabetes and minimize the progression of complications. Appointments were made with the diabetes educator and dietician during the same week. Dr. Grady informed Mrs. Johnson that in the future, he would like her to make an appointment with an ophthalmologist for a dilated eye exam, a podiatrist for foot care, and a counselor to discuss her feelings related to diagnosis of a chronic disease and her concerns related to her graduate studies. Dr. Grady provided Mrs. Johnson with his e-mail address and encouraged her to use it if she had questions related to the treatment of her diabetes. A follow-up appointment was made for 3 months later.

(Continued on page 66)

(Continued from page 65)

Dr. Grady informed Mrs. Johnson that he was ordering a baseline electrocardiogram (EKG); laboratory values for total cholesterol, LDL, HDL, and triglycerides; and a Hemoglobin A1C. He instructed her on how to dial into the 24-hour automatic recorded information system to obtain her laboratory results.

After the visit, Dr. Grady entered his physician notes into the medical record on his personal digital assistant (PDA). He downloaded the medical record into the diabetes registry, which allowed team members access to current data so they were able to individualize the treatment and education plan for Mrs. Johnson before her next visit.

During her visit with Mrs. Johnson, the diabetes educator reviewed the physiology of diabetes and taught her how to use the glucometer. She had the patient complete a return demonstration so she could answer questions related to the use of the monitor. The diabetes educator assisted Mrs. Johnson in setting a self-management goal of documenting her daily blood sugar levels. She provided Mrs. Johnson with a patient diary to document her meals and blood sugar levels and encouraged her to bring it on return medical visits. She elicited questions from Mrs. Johnson and was able to address the patient's concerns related to her roles as wife and mother. She encouraged Mrs. Johnson to bring her husband to the next visit so his questions and concerns could be addressed. She directed Mrs. Johnson to a website that provided online interactive diabetes classes. In addition, the diabetes educator referred Mrs. Johnson to a chat room that would allow her to communicate with other individuals with diabetes. She provided Mrs. Johnson with her e-mail address for questions and scheduled a follow-up appointment for 1 month later. A team meeting was also scheduled to review Mrs. Johnson's treatment plan and address family members' educational needs and concerns.

The dietician conducted a dietary evaluation and provided nutritional education. She discussed the relationship between food intake and blood sugar levels. When the dietician discussed the importance of exercise, Mrs. Johnson said she wanted to start an exercise program. The dietician assisted her with the development of a self-management goal in which she exercised three times a week for 30 minutes. The dietician also provided Mrs. Johnson with her e-mail address and referred her to a website that provided information on how to make lifestyle changes. A follow-up appointment was scheduled for Mrs. Johnson for 1 month later. The dietician encouraged her to have family members attend future appointments so their questions or concerns could be addressed.

and support according to the recommended standards of care. The team members, including Mrs. Johnson and her husband, met to communicate and coordinate the treatment plan.

Third, the health care professionals *employed evidenced-based practice*. Health professionals frequently expect newly diagnosed diabetics to change multiple behaviors to decrease their risk of complications. Patients often fail at self-management because they are overwhelmed by the number of changes. In accordance with the current literature, the diabetes educator and dietician each had Mrs. Johnson choose one basic self-management goal. They provided her with the information and tools necessary to be successful, and then on her follow-up visits, they reviewed her progress.

Fourth, the team *applied quality improvement* in the provision of care through use of the diabetes registry. Key outcome measures were tracked for individual patients, a subpopulation, or the general registry population. At Mrs. Johnson's next appointment, health care providers will print out a record that displays data and graphs of visits and care provided for the past 6 months. Doing so allows providers and patients to note trends. In addition, care reminders can be printed out and given to health care providers to remind them of needed services, or a letter can be sent to the patient as a reminder for care.

Finally, health care providers *utilized informatics* as a way to communicate and manage Mrs. Johnson's diabetes care. All the health care providers used PDAs to input data into the diabetes registry so they had continual access to updated information. Mrs. Johnson was able to obtain results of her EKG and laboratory tests from an automatic recorded information system. If she had questions related to diabetes and self-management, she had e-mail access to her health care team. In addition, she was encouraged to seek out current diabetes information on the Web while obtaining support from others with diabetes through a chat room.

Conclusion

In conclusion, the committee stresses that narrowing of the quality chasm can be realized, at least in part, by reforming health professions education:

- **For health professionals, there is a set of core competencies that can advance adherence to the rules of a redesigned health care system as envisioned in the Quality Chasm report: provide patient-centered care, work in interdisciplinary teams, employ evidence-based practice, apply quality improvement, and utilize informatics.**

- **The extent to which current health professionals are implementing these competency areas does not meet the health care needs of the American public.**

References

ABIM Foundation. 2002. Medical professionalism in the new millennium: A physician charter. *Annals of Internal Medicine* 136 (3):243-46.

Agency for Healthcare Research and Quality. 2002. "Evidence-based Practice Centers." Online. Available at http://www.ahrq.gov/clinic/epcix.htm [accessed Dec. 1, 2002].

American Association of Medical Colleges. 2001. "Medical School Objectives Project." Online. Available at http://www.aamc.org/meded/msop/start.htm [accessed Sept., 2002].

American Cancer Society. 2002. "No Matter Who You Are. We Can Help." Online. Available at http://www.cancer.org/docroot/home/index.asp [accessed Dec. 1, 2002].

American College of Physicians. 2002. "ACP Journal Club." Online. Available at http://www.acpjc.org/shared/purpose_and_procedure.htm [accessed Dec., 2002].

Amsterdam, J.T., D.K. Wagner, and L.F. Rose. 1980. Interdisciplinary training: Hospital dental general practice/emergency medicine. *Annals of Emergency Medicine* 9 (6):310-313.

Bader, S.A., and R.M. Braude. 1998. "Patient informatics": Creating new partnerships in medical decision making. *Academic Medicine* 73 (4):408-11.

Balas, E.A. 2001. Information systems can prevent errors and improve quality. *Journal of the American Medical Informatics Association* 8 (4):398-99.

Baldwin, D. 1996. Some historical notes on interdisciplinary and interprofessional education and practice in health care in the U.S. *Journal of Interprofessional Care* 10:173-87.

Batalden, P., D. Leach, S. Swing, H. Dreyfus, and S. Dreyfus. 2002. General competencies and accreditation in graduate medical education. *Health Affairs* 21 (5):103-11.

Bates, D.W., L.L. Leape, D.J. Cullen, N. Laird, L.A. Petersen, J.M. Teich, E. Burdick, M. Hickey, S. Kleefield, B. Shea, M. Vander Vliet, and D.L. Seger. 1998. Effect of computerized physician order entry and a team intervention on prevention of serious medication errors. *Journal of American Medical Association* 280 (15): 1311-16.

Bates, D.W., J.M. Teich, J. Lee, et al. 1999. The impact of computerized physician order entry on medication error prevention. *Journal of the American Medical Informatics Association* 6 (4):313-21.

Benbassat, J., D. Pilpel, and M. Tidhar. 1998. Patients preferences for participation in clinical decision making: A review of published surveys. *Behavorial Medicine* 24 (2):81-88.

Benner, P. 1982. Issues in competency-based testing. *Nursing Outlook* 30 (5):303-9.

Berwick, D.M. 1996. A primer on leading the improvement of systems. *British Medical Journal* 312 (7031):619-22.

Berwick, D.M., A. Enthoven, and J.P. Bunker. 1992. Quality management in the NHS: The doctors role--II. *British Medical Journal* 304 (6822):304-8.

Blendon, R.J., C.M. DesRoches, M. Brodie, J.M. Benson, A.B. Rosen, E. Schneider, D.E. Altman, K. Zapert, M.J. Herrmann, and A.E. Steffenson. 2002. Views of practicing physicians and the public on medical errors. *N Engl J Med* 347 (24):1933-40.

Blumenthal, D., and A.M. Epstein. 1996. The role of physicians in the future of quality management- part six of six. *New England Journal of Medicine* 335 (17):1328-32.

Blumenthal, D., and C.M. Kilo. 1998. A report card on continuous quality improvement. *Milbank Q* 76 (4):625-48, 511.

Blumenthal, D. 1997. The future of quality measurement and management in a transforming health care system. *Journal of the American Medical Association* 278 (19):1622-25.

Bluml, B.M., L.R. Copeland, B. LeTourneau, M.O. Mundinger, R. Nelson, and U. Reinhardt. 1999. Health care trends, Part 2. The new health care team. Panel discussion. *Physician Executive* 25 (4):67-75.

Bodenheimer, T., E.H. Wagner, and K. Grumbach. 2002. Improving primary care for patients with chronic illness. *Journal of the American Medical Association* 288 (14):1775-9.

Brady, M., J.D. Leuner, J.P. Bellack, R.S. Loquist, P. F. Cipriano, and E.H. O'Neil. 2001. A proposed framework for differentiating the 21 PEW competencies by level of nursing

education. *Nursing & Health Care Perspectives* 22 (1):30-35.

Brennan, T.A. 1998. The role of regulation in quality improvement. *Milbank Quarterly* 76 (4):709-31, 512.

Brotherton, S.E., F.A. Simon, and S.I. Etzel. 2001. U.S. Graduate Medical Education, 2000-2001. *Journal of American Medical Association.* 286 (9):1056-60.

Burl, J.B., A. Bonner, M. Rao, and A.M. Khan. 1998. Geriatric nurse practitioners in long-term care: Demonstration of effectiveness in managed care. *Journal American Geriatrics Society* 46 (4):506-10.

Cain, M. M., R. Mittman, J. Sarasohn-Kahn, and J. C. Wayne. 2000. *Health e-People: The Online Consumer Experience.* Oakland, CA: Institute for the Future, California Health Care Foundation.

Center for the Advancement of Pharmaceutical Education [CAPE] Advisory Panel on Educational Outcomes. 1998. "Educational Outcomes." Online. Available at http://www. aacp.org/Docs/MainNavigation/ Resources/3933_edoutcom.doc? DocTypeID=4&TrackID=&VID=1&CID=410& DID=366 [accessed Dec. 10, 2002].

Centers for Medicaid and Medicare Services. 2002. "HIPPA Insurance Reform." Online. Available at http://cms.hhs.gov/hipaa/hipaa1/default.asp [accessed 2002].

Chassin, M.R. 1998. Is health care ready for Six Sigma quality? *Milbank Quarterly* 76 (4):565-91, 510.

Cochrane Collaboration. 2001. "Cochrane Brochure." Online. Available at http://www. cochrane.org/cochrane/cc-broch.htm [accessed Sept. 20, 2002].

Cooley, K.A., P.S. Frame, and S.W. Eberly. 1999. After the grant runs out. Long-term provider health maintenance compliance using a computer-based tracking system. *Archives in Family Medicine* 8 (1):13-17.

Cooper, B. S. and E. Fishman. 2003. *The Interdisciplinry Team in the Management of Chronic Conditions: Has its Time Come?* Baltimore, MD: Partnership for Solutions.

Curley, C., J.E. McEachern, and T. Speroff. 1998.

A firm trial of interdisciplinary rounds on the inpatient medical wards: an intervention designed using continuous quality improvement. *Medical Care* 36 (8 Suppl):AS4-12.

Davidoff, F. 1999. In the teeth of the evidence. The curious case of evidence-based medicine. *The Mount Sinai Journal of Medicine* 66 (2):75-83.

Davidoff, F. and V. Florance. 2000. The informationist: A new health profession? *Annals of Internal Medicine* 132 (12):996-98.

Denehy, J. 1998. Integrating nursing outcomes classification in nursing education. *Journal of Nursing Care Quality* 12 (5):73-84.

Department of Health and Human Services, H.R.a.S. A.B.o.P.H.c. 1998. Health Center Program Expectations. *Bureau of Primary Health Care Policy Information Notice: 98-23.*

DiCenso, A., N. Cullum, and D. Ciliska. 1998. Implementing evidence-based nursing: Some misconceptions [editorial]. *Evidence-Based Nursing* 1:38-40.

Donabedian, A. 1980. *Explorations in Quality Assessment and Monitoring, Volume 1: The Definition of Quality and Approaches to Its Assessment.* Ann Arbor, Michigan: Health Adminsitration Press.

Epstein, R.M., and E.M. Hundert. 2002. Defining and assessing professional competence. *Journal of the American Medical Association* 287 (2):226-35.

Evans, R.S., S.L. Pestotnik, D.C. Classen, T.P. Clemmer, L.K. Weaver, J.F. Orme, Jr., J.F. Lloyd, and J.P. Burke. 1998. A computer-assisted management program for antibiotics and other anti-infective agents. *New England Journal of Medicine* 338 (4):232-38.

Evers, G. 2001. Naming nursing: Evidence-based nursing. *Nursing Diagnosis* 12 (4):137-42.

Ferlie, E.B., and S.M. Shortell. 2001. Improving the quality of health care in the United Kingdom and the United States: A framework for change. *Milbank Quarterly* 79 (2):281-315.

Gambrill, E. 1999. Evidence-based clinical practice. *Journal of Behavior Therapy and Experimental Psychiatry* 30 (1):1-14.

Gerteis, M., S. Edgman-Levitan, J. Daley, and T. Delbanco, editors. 1993. *Through the Patient Eyes.* Vol. San Francisco, CA: Josey-Bass.

Gifford, A.L., D.D. Laurent, V.M. Gonzales, et al. 1998. Pilot randomized trial of education to improve self-management skills of men with symptomatic HIV/AIDS. *Journal of Acquired Immune Deficiency Syndromes and Human Retrovirology* 18 (2):136-44.

Goldberg, H.I., R.A. Deyo, V.M. Taylor, A.D. Cheadle, D.A. Conrad, J.D. Loeser, P.J. Heagerty, and P. Diehr. 2001. Can evidence change the rate of back surgery? A randomized trial of community-based education. *Effective Clinical Practice* 4 (3):95-104.

Grad, R., A.C. Macaulay, and M. Warner. 2001. Teaching evidence-based medical care: Description and evaluation. *Family Medicine* 33 (8):602-6.

Green, P.L. 1998. Improving clinical effectiveness in an integrated care delivery system. *Journal for Healthcare Quality* 20 (6):4-8; quiz 9, 48.

Griffin Hospital. 2002. "Griffin News--The Latest News About Griffin." Online. Available at http://www.griffinhealth.org/news/ [accessed Oct. 12, 2002].

Grol, R. 2001. Improving the quality of medical care: Building bridges among professional pride, payer profit, and patient satisfaction. *Journal of the American Medical Association* 286 (20):2578-85.

Guyatt, G.H., R.B. Haynes, R.Z. Jaeschke, D.J. Cook, L. Green, C.D. Naylor, M. Wilson, and W.S. Richardson. 2000. Users guide to the medical literature: XXV. Evidence-based medicine: Principles for applying the users guides to patient care. *Journal of American Medical Association* 284 (10):1290-1296.

Hall, P., and L. Weaver. 2001. Interdisciplinary education and teamwork: A long and winding road. *Medical Education* 35 (9):867-75.

Halpern, R., M.Y. Lee, P.R. Boulter, and R.R. Phillips. 2001. A synthesis of nine major reports on physicians competencies for the emerging practice environment. *Academic Medicine* 76 (6):606-15.

Hart, J.T. 1995. Clinical and economic consequences of patients as producers. *Journal of Public Health Medicine* 17 (4):383-86.

Haynes, R.B. 2002. What kind of evidence is it that evidence-based medicine advocates want health care providers and consumers to pay attention to? *BMC Health Serv Res* 2 (1):3.

Health Disparities Collaboratives. 2001. "Changing Practice, Changing Lives." Online. Available at http://www.healthdisparities.net/index.html [accessed Fall, 2002].

Helmreich, R.L. 2000. On error management: Lessons from aviation. *British Medical Journal* 320 (7237):781-85.

Henbest, R.J., and M. Stewart. 1990. Patient-centredness in the consultation. 2: Does it really make a difference? *Family Practice* 7 (1):28-33.

Higgs, J.P., A.M. Burn, and M.M. Jones. 2001. Integrating clinical reasoning and evidence-based practice. *Association of Critical-Care Nurses Clinical Issues: Advanced Practice in Acute & Critical Care* 12 (4):482-90.

Holman, W.L., R.M. Allman, M. Sansom, C.I. Kiefe, E.D. Peterson, K.J. Anstrom, S.S. Sankey, S.G. Hubbard, and R.G. Sherrill. 2001. Alabama coronary artery bypass grafting project: Results of a statewide quality improvement initiative. *Journal of the American Medical Association* 285 (23):3003-10.

Houston, T.K., and H.E. Ehrenberger. 2001. The potential of consumer health informatics. *Seminars in Oncology Nursing* 17 (1):41-47.

Hunt, D.L., B.R. Haynes, S. Harna, and K. Smith. 1998. Effects of computer-based clinical decision support systems on physician performance and patient outcomes. *Journal of American Medical Association* 280 (15):1339-46.

Institute for Healthcare Improvement, and National Coalition on Health Care. 2002. *Accelerating Change Today A.C.T for Americas Health--Curing the System.*, Schoeni, P.Q., ed. Boston, MA: National Coalition on Health Care and the Institute for Healthcare Improvement.

Institute for the Future. 2000. *Health and Health Care, 2010: The Forecast, The Challenge Based on 1998 Data Provided by the Department of Finance, State of California.* San Francisco, CA: Institute for the Future.

Institute of Medicine. 1990. *Medicare: A Strategy for Quality Assurance: Executive Summary IOM Committee to Design a Strategy for Quality Review and Assurance in Medicare.* Washington: National Academy Press.

———. 1997. *The Computer-Based Patient Record: An Essential Technology for Health Care.* Revised edition. Richard S. Dick, Elaine B. Steen , and Don E. Detmer, eds. Washington, DC: National Academy Press.

———. 2000. *To Err Is Human: Building a Safer Health System.* Linda T. Kohn, Janet M. Corrigan, and Molla S. Donaldson, eds. Washington, DC: National Academy Press.

———. 2001. *Crossing the Quality Chasm: A New Health System for the 21st Century.* Washington, DC: National Academy Press.

———. 2002. *Leadership By Example.* Washington, DC: National Academies Press.

Jadad, A.R., and R.B. Haynes. 1998. The Cochrane Collaboration--advances and challenges in improving evidence-based decision making. *Medical Decision Making* 18 (1):2-9; discussion 16-8.

Kaplan, S.H., S. Greenfield, and J.E. Ware, Jr. 1989. Assessing the effects of physician-patient interactions on the outcomes of chronic disease. *Medical Care* 27 (3 Suppl):S110-27.

Khuri, S.F., J. Daley, and W.G. Henderson. 2002. The comparative assessment and improvement of quality of surgical care in the Department of Veterans Affairs. *Archives of Surgery* 137 (1):20-27.

Kiefe, C.I., J.J. Allison, O.D. Williams, S.D. Person, M.T. Weaver, and N.W. Weissman. 2001. Improving quality improvement using achievable benchmarks for physician feedback: A randomized controlled trial. *Journal of the American Medical Association* 285 (22):2871-9.

Lang, N.M. 1999. Discipline-based approaches to evidence-based practice: a view from nursing. *Joint Commission Journal on Quality Improvement* 25 (10):539-44.

Lenburg, C., R. Redman, and P. Hinton. 1999. "Competency Assessment: Methods for Development and Implementation in Nursing Education." Online. Available at in cabinet [accessed Mar. 19, 2002].

Lewin, S.A., Z.C. Skea, V. Entwistle, M. Zwarenstein, and J. Dick. 2001. Interventions for providers to promote a patient-centred approach in clinical consultations (Cochrane Review). *Cochrane Database System Review*

4:CD003267.

Lobach, D.F., and W.E. Hammond. 1997. Computerized decision support based on a clinical practice guideline improves compliance with care standards. *American Journal of Medicine* 102 (1):89-98.

Lorig, K.R., D.S. Sobel, P.L. Ritter, D. Laurent, and M. Hobbs. 2001. Effect of a self-management program on patients with chronic disease. *Effective Clinical Practice* 4 (6):256-62.

Lorig, K.R., D.S. Sobel, A.L. Steward, et al. 1999. Evidence suggesting that a chronic disease self-management program can improve health status while reducing hospitalization: A randomized trial. *Medical Care* 37 (1):5-14.

Luciano, L. 2000. A government health system leads the way. *Accelerating Change Today A.C.T. for America's Health--Reducing Medical Errors and Improving Patient Safety.* Institute for Healthcare Improvement, and National Coalition on Health Care. Boston, MA: Institute for Healthcare Improvement, National Coalition on Health Care.

MacDonald, K., J. Case, and J. Metzger. 2001. *E-Encounters.* Oakland, CA: California Health Foundation.

Mallow, G.E., and F. Gilje. 1999. Technology-based nursing education: Overview and call for further dialogue. [see comments]. [Review] [36 refs]. *Journal of Nursing Education* 38 (6):248-51.

Masys, D., D. Baker, A. Butros, and K.E. Cowles. 2002. Giving patients access to their medical records via the internet: The PCASSO experience. *Journal of the American Medical Informatics Association* 9 (2):181-91.

Masys, D.R. 1998. Advances in information technology. Implications for medical education. *Western Journal of Medicine* 168 (5):341-47.

Masys, D.R., P.F. Brennan, J.G. Ozbolt, M. Corn, and E.H. Shortliffe. 2000. Are medical informatics and nursing informatics distinct disciplines? The 1999 ACMI debate. *Journal of American Medical Information Association* 7 (3):304-12.

Mazurek, B. 2002. Strategies for overcoming barriers in implementing evidence-based practice. *Periatric Nursing* 28 (2):159-61.

McCulloch, D.K., M.J. Price, M. Hindmarsh, and E. H. Wagner. 1998. A population-based approach to diabetes management in a primary care setting: Early results and lessons learned. *Effective Clinical Practice* 1 (1):12-22.

McDonough, R.P. and W.R. Doucette. 2001. Dynamics of pharmaceutical care: Developing collaborative working relationships between pharmacists and physicians. *Journal of American Pharmaceutical Association* 41 (5):682-92.

Mead, N., and P. Bower. 2000. Patient-centredness: A conceptual framework and review of the empirical literature. *Social Science Medicine* 51 (7):1087-110.

Mehta, R.H., S. Das, T.T. Tsai, E. Nolan, G. Kearly, and K.A. Eagle. 2000. Quality improvement initiative and its impact on the management of patients with acute myocardial infarction. *Archives of Medicine* 160 (20):3057-62.

Mehta, R.H., C.K. Montoye, M. Gallogly, P. Baker, A. Blount, J. Faul, C. Roychoudhury, S. Borzak, S. Fox, M. Franklin, M. Freundl, E. Kline-Rogers, T. LaLonde, M. Orza, R. Parrish, M. Satwicz, M.J. Smith, P. Sobotka, S. Winston, A.A. Riba, and K.A. Eagle. 2002. Improving quality of care for acute myocardial infarction: The Guidelines Applied in Practice (GAP) Initiative. *Journal of American Medical Association* 287 (10):1269-76.

Meryn, S. 1998. Improving communication skills: To carry coals to... *Medical Teacher* 20 (4):331-37.

Mycek, S. 2001. Good fortune. Griffin Hospital gets outstanding grades in both employee and patient satisfaction. *Trustee* 54 (7):20-24, 1.

National Committee on Vital and Health Statistics. 2000. "Uniform Data Standards for Patient Medical Record Information." Online. Available at http://ncvhs.hhs.gov/hipaa000706.pdf [accessed Aug. 30, 2002].

National Institutes of Health. 2002. "National Institute of Health Web site." Online. Available at www.nih.gov [accessed May 13, 2002].

National Library of Medicine. 2002. "PubMed Overview." Online. Available at http://www. ncbi.nlm.nih.gov/entrez/query/static/overview. html#Introduction [accessed Dec. 1, 2002].

NHS Centre for Review and Dissemination. 2002.

"Database of Abstracts of Review of Effectiveness (DARE)." Online. Available at http://agatha.york.ac.uk/darehp.htm [accessed Dec. 1, 2002].

OConnor, G.T., S.K. Plume, E.M. Olmstead, J.R. Morton, C.T. Maloney, W.C. Nugent, F. Hernandez, Jr. , R. Clough, B.J. Leavitt, L.H. Coffin, C.A. Marrin, D. Wennberg, J.D. Birkmeyer, D.C. Charlesworth, D.J. Malenka, H.B. Quinton, and J.F. Kasper. 1996. A regional intervention to improve the hospital mortality associated with coronary artery bypass graft surgery. The Northern New England Cardiovascular Disease Study Group. *Journal of the American Medical Association* 275 (11):841-46.

Oliver Goldsmith. 2000. "Culturally competent health care. *The Permanente Journal.* 4(1)." Online. Available at http://www. kaiserpermanente.org/medicine/permjournal/ winter00pj/frcompetent.html [accessed Nov. 1, 2002].

ONeil, E. H. and the Pew Health Professions Commission. 1998. *Recreating health professional practice for a new century - The fourth report of the PEW health professions Commission.* San Francisco, CA: Pew Health Professions Commission.

Overhage, J.M., W.M. Tierney, X.H. Zhou, and C.J. McDonald. 1997. A randomized trial of corollary orders to prevent errors of omission. *Journal of the American Medical Informatics Association* 4 (5):364-75.

Pew Health Professions Commission. 1995. *Critical Challenges: Revitalizing the Health Professions for the Twenty-First Century .* San Francisco, CA: UCSF Center for the Health Professions:

Raymond, B., and C. Dold. 2002. *Clinical Information Systems: Achieving the Vision.* Oakland: Kaiser Permanente Institute for Health Policy .

Rebillot, K. 2000. Taking Medication Errors Head On. *Accelerating Change Today A.C.T for Americas Health--Reducing Medical Errors and Improving Patient Safety.* Institute for Healthcare Improvement, and National Coalition on Health Care. Boston, MA: Institute for Healthcare Improvement, National Coalition on Health Care.

Reese, D.J., and M.A. Sontag. 2001. Successful interprofessional collaboration on the hospice team. *Health & Social Work* 26 (3):167-75.

Robert Wood Johnson Foundation. 2002. "Improving Chronic Illness Care." Online. Available at www.improvingchroniccare.org [accessed Oct., 2002].

Rosswurm, M.A., and J.H. Larrabee. 1999. A model for change to evidence-based practice. *Image Journal of Nursing Scholarship* 31 (4):317-22.

Roter, D.L., J.A. Hall, D.E. Kern, L.R. Barker, K.A. Cole, and R.P. Roca. 1995. Improving physicians interviewing skills and reducing patients emotional distress. A randomized clinical trial. *Archives of Internal Medicine* 155 (17):1877-84.

Saba, V.K. 2001. Nursing informatics: Yesterday, today and tomorrow. *International Nursing Review* 48 (3):177-87.

Saranto, K., and H. Leino-Kilpi. 1997. Computer literacy in nursing: Developing the information technology syllabus in nursing education. *Journal of Advanced Nursing* 25 (2):377-85.

Schuster, M.A., E.A. McGlynn, and R.H. Brook. 1998. How good is the quality of health care in the United States? *Milbank Quarterly* 76 (4):517-63, 509.

Shortell, S.M., C.L. Bennett, and G.R. Byck. 1998. Assessing the impact of continuous quality improvement on clinical practice: What it will take to accelerate progress. *Milbank Quarterly* 76 (4):593-624, 510.

Shortell, S. 1994. The performance of intensive care units. *Medical Care* 32(5):508-25.

Silver, M.P., and J.A. Antonow. 2000. Reducing medication errors in hospitals: A peer review organization collaboration. *Joint Commission Journal on Quality Improvement* 26 (6):332-40.

Sinclair, M., and J. Gardner. 1999. Planning for information technology: Key skills in nurse education. *Journal of Advanced Medicine* 30 (6):1441-50.

Stewart, M. 2001. Towards a global definition of patient centered care. *British Medical Journal* 322 (7284):444-45.

Stewart, M., J.B. Brown, H. Boon, J. Galajda, L. Meredith, and M. Sangster. 1999. Evidence on patient-doctor communication. *Cancer*

Prevention Control 3 (1):25-30.

Straus, S.E., and D.L. Sackett. 1998. Using research findings in clinical practice. *British Medical Journal* 317 (7154):339-42.

Superio-Cabuslay, E., M.M. Ward, and K.R. Lorig. 1996. Patient education interventions in osteoarthritis and rheumatoid arthritis: A meta-analytic comparison with nonsteroidal anti-inflammatory drug treatment. *Arthritis Care Research* 9 (4):292-301.

Unutzer, J.M.M., L.M.M. Rubenstein, W.J.M. Katon , L.P. Tang, N.P. Duan, I.T.M. Lagomasino, and K.B.M.M. Wells. 2001. Two-year effects of quality improvement programs on medication management for depression. *Archives of General Psychiatry* 58 (10):935-42.

Von Korff, M., J. Gruman, J. Schaefer, S.J. Curry, and E.H. Wagner. 1997. Collaborative management of chronic illness. *Annals of Internal Medicine* 127 (12):1097-102.

Von Korff, M., J.E. Moore, K.R. Lorig, et al. 1998. A randomized trial of a lay person-led self-management group intervention for back pain patients in primary care. *Spine* 23 (23):2608-51.

Wagner, E.H. 1998. Chronic disease management: What will it take to improve care for chronic illness? *Effective Clinical Practice.* 1 (1):2-4.

Wagner, E.H., B.T. Austin, C. Davis, M. Hindmarsh, J. Schaefer, and A. Bonomi. 2001. Improving chronic illness care: Translating evidence into action. *Health Affairs* 20 (6):64-78.

Wagner, E.H., B.T. Austin, and M. Von Korff. 1996. Organizing care for patients with chronic illness. [Review] [121 refs]. *Milbank Quarterly.* 74 (4):511-44.

Wagner, E.H., R.E. Glasgow, C. Davis, A.E. Bonomi, L. Provost, D. McCulloch, P. Carver, and C. Sixta. 2001. Quality improvement in chronic illness care: A collaborative approach. *Joint Commission Journal on Quality Improvement* 27 (2):63-80.

Wagner, E.H. 2000. The role of patient care teams in chronic disease management. *British Medical Journal* 320 (7234):569-72.

Walshe, K., and T.G. Rundall. 2001. Evidence-based management: From theory to practice in health care. *Milbank Quarterly* 79 (3):429-57, IV-V.

Weeks, W.B., P.D. Mills, R.S. Dittus, D.C. Aron, and P.B. Batalden. 2001. Using an improvement model to reduce adverse drug events in VA facilities. *Joint Commission Journal on Quality Improvement* 27 (5):243-54.

Weingart, S.N. 1996. House officer education and organizational obstacles to quality improvement. *Joint Commission Journal on Quality Improvement* 22 (9):640-646.

Wu, S., and A. Green. 2000. *Projection of Chronic Illness Prevalence and Cost Inflation.* California: RAND Health.

Zielstorff, R. 1998. Characteristics of a good nursing nomenclature from an informatics perspective. *Online Journal of Issues in Nursing*

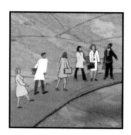

Chapter 4
Current Educational Activities in the Core Competencies

This chapter reviews current undergraduate and graduate educational activities for medicine, nursing, pharmacy, and selected allied health professions with respect to the core competencies outlined in Chapter 3: provide patient-centered care, employ evidence-based practice, work in interdisciplinary teams, apply quality improvement, and utilize informatics. The focus is on what, how, and when health professionals are taught these competencies in academic programs. There is broad variation in this regard. Some of these competencies are intrinsic to the historical vision of certain professions, while others are inadequately addressed in the educational programs of any of the professions. The chapter concludes with a discussion of how educational institutions are moving toward an outcome-based education approach to ensure that students can demonstrate such competencies upon graduation, and a review of the issues surrounding this approach.

The committee obtained information published in the professional literature and supplemented these published descriptions by soliciting input from educational institutions The committee notes that there are few rigorous evaluations of educational interventions in the health professions. Indeed, the lack of evidence-based education is an issue that the committee decided to address with a recommendation and that a working group at the summit deemed important to address (see Appendix C). Studies examining the effect of education in any quantifiable manner come largely from medical education, which accounts for the predominance of references related to medical education in this chapter. In discussing preparation in the five competencies, the professions are addressed in order of the extent of available evidence: medicine, nursing, pharmacy, and allied health.

Provide Patient-Centered Care

In general, comprehensive attention to patient-centered care in medical education is lacking. The dominant biomedical model of practice, whereby patients are viewed in terms of signs and symptoms, remains a large barrier to redressing this need (Mead and Bower, 2000). Though efforts to teach patient-centered care, however defined, are increasingly being advocated and incorporated into the training of physicians (Lewin et al., 2001), such efforts are regarded as ad hoc and are often not ascribed significant value, energy, and financial resources (Flores et al., 2000; Malloch et al., 2000). Shared and informed decision making with patients needs greater emphasis in medical education. One survey of medical students and residents revealed that over 90 percent of respondents believed physicians should have greater input in decisions than patients; as training and experience increased beyond medical school, there was an increased tendency toward a belief in physician-only decision making (Beisecker et al., 1996).

Medical students also are not adequately prepared for promoting prevention and healthy lifestyles with patients. Although an expert panel convened by the Association of Teachers of Preventive Medicine proposed a curricular requirement "of making preventive medicine an integral part of the education, training, and practice of physicians" (Collins et al., 1991:307), the integration of disease and illness prevention and wellness into medical education has largely not been achieved (Garr et al., 2000; Heller et al., 2000; Institute of Medicine, 1988; Pomrehn et al., 2000). Indeed, given the tradition in medicine of overwork, sleep deprivation, and neglect of one's own wellness, medical students and residents cannot even serve as good examples for patients of healthy lifestyles and wellness.

Medical education has recently placed more emphasis on enhancing patient–clinician communication, and such efforts have been shown to increase patient satisfaction and improve patient outcomes (Halpern et al., 2001; Henbest and Stewart, 1990; Langewitz et al., 1998; Lewin et al., 2001; Lipkin, 1996; Smith et al., 1995; Swick et al., 1999). However, there is broad variation in the content and evaluation of communication courses. The American Association of Medical Colleges (AAMC) has begun to address this lack of uniformity by developing communication competencies through its Medical School Objective Project (American Association of Medical Colleges, 2000).

Nurses have long been taught to focus on the patient's needs, the family, or in some cases, a clinically defined population group. On balance, they are educated to use preventive and health-promoting interventions, to counsel and communicate with patients, to apply community and behavioral interventions, and to be highly sensitive to the needs of individuals (Allen, 2000; Milio, 2002; O'Neil and the Pew Health Professions Commission, 1998). However, the realities of the day-to-day practice environment and systems design often constrain opportunities to utilize this knowledge fully (Peterson, 2001). Further, some worry that there are major differences among nursing programs with regard to educational preparedness in competencies associated with population-focused care, health protection, and promotion and prevention (Institute of Medicine, 1995).

In the last decade, pharmacists have reformulated their vision of the profession, shifting from an orientation primarily toward the dispensing of drugs to a greater focus on pharmaceutical care, an approach designed to promote health; prevent disease; and assess, monitor, initiate, and modify medication use to ensure that drug therapy regimens are safe and effective (American Pharmacuetical Association, 2002). The result has been a widespread curricular change in pharmacy education during the last decade to better prepare graduates for this new mission (American Association of Colleges of Pharmacy Commission to Implement Change in Pharmaceutical Education, 1993; Center for the Advancement of Pharmaceutical Education [CAPE] Advisory Panel on Educational Outcomes, 1998; Pharmacy Deans Task Force on Professionalism, 2000). In these reform efforts, considerable emphasis has been placed on a revision of curricula to include more service learning opportunities and education of students in new communication and health promotion and disease prevention competencies (Murawski et al., 1999). Though changes have been substantial, a recent survey of pharmacy faculty revealed that training in communication skills is irregular and not well developed in some schools (Beardsley, 2001).

Prevention and health promotion, as well as shared decision making with patients, are intrinsic to the vision of a number of allied health professions, including dental hygienist, registered dietician, physical therapist, and occupational therapist, and the educational preparation and curricula for these professions reflect this fact. However, the Association of Schools of Allied Health Professions and the National Commission on Allied Health (Health Resources and Services Administration, 1999), citing allied health professionals' frequent contact with patients and their relative lack of preparation in this area, have suggested that allied health curricula be strengthened further to include communication and patient and family education.

Being competent in providing patient-centered care includes easing pain and providing comfort to patients who need it. These skills are particularly important in end-of-life care. Yet review commissions have found that pain management is not sufficiently addressed in the education of all the health professions to meet the needs of the American people (Institute of Medicine, 2001; 2002b). In one survey, the authors reviewed postgraduate medical training programs on the care of seriously ill and dying patients and found that the majority included no training in pain assessment and management (Weissman and Block, 2002). And while nurses have been central in the development of the international hospice movement, specific educational opportunities for nurses in pain management are still rare (Institute of Medicine, 2002b). The American Association of Colleges of Nursing has concluded that "end-of-life education and training is inconsistent at best and sometimes completely neglected within nursing curricula" (American Association of Colleges of Nursing, 2002:1)

Understanding the patient's values and experience outside of the hospital necessitates cross-cultural awareness and competence. However, there is little documentation of the extent to which cross-cultural issues are covered in the education of health professionals (Institute of Medicine, 2002a). Summit participants stressed the need to develop cultural competency standards to promote better understanding of and communication with diverse populations, as well as increased education in community settings in the form of home visits and community-based partnerships with schools. Participants emphasized the importance of involving patients and their families in all aspects of the educational process, including having them rate student performance in providing care, holding more clinical discussions at bedside, videotaping encounters between students and patients, and using patient focus groups to provide feedback on performance. Research supports the view that these techniques greatly enhance patient satisfaction and facilitate better student performance with patients (Branch, 2000; Branch et al., 2001; Chisholm and Wade, 1999; Eyler et al., 2001; Gerteis et al., 1993; Maguire et al., 1996; Novack et al., 1999; Self et al., 1998). Box 4-1 presents some examples of effective education in patient-centered care.

Box 4-1. Education in Patient-Centered Care: Selected Examples

The **Auburn University School of Nursing** converted in 2000 from a quarter system to a semester system. This conversion became a catalyst for an overall curriculum change focused on service learning. The idea that nursing is a partnership with the client that can take place in any setting became the guiding vision for the change. All of the major clinical courses were revised to include community health experiences, such as assessments of families and communities, physical assessment of clients at their work, and health promotion activities. Validation of certain students' skills takes place not at school, but in community settings as diverse as public housing facilities, day care centers, industry work sites, and assisted living facilities. Students follow patients through admission, discharge, and home care, applying case management principles throughout (Hamner and Wilder, 2001; Marvel et al., 1999).

The biopsychosocial model of education of the **University of Rochester School of Medicine** emphasizes the essential interrelationships among biological, psychological, and social forces in health and illness. The model includes sessions on communication with patients and population-based care, as well as exercises in which students explore influences of their families and cultures on their attitudes and motivations by sharing family trees and writing personal illness narratives. Practical exercises that teach students how to communicate with patients about death and dying, violence, race, culture, and disability are also employed (Novack et al., 1999).

University of Massachusetts Medical School, **New York University School of Medicine**, and **Case Western Reserve University School of Medicine** are part of a 4-year initiative funded by the **Macy Foundation** to define fundamental competencies in health communication, develop curriculum that is based on these competencies, formulate objective evaluation techniques to measure the communication competence of students and residents, and create and disseminate a national model for faculty development in health communication. As a condition of their participation, the three institutions have agreed to the goal of integrating health communication into all 4 years of the medical school curriculum. The results of this effort will be used in the development of a Macy Scholars in Health Education program that will both educate faculty in the knowledge and skills needed to pursue careers in health communication and enable them to bring new communication initiatives into their medical institutions (Bloom, 1989).

White Memorial Medical Center Family Practice Residency Program in Los Angeles, California, serves the local community of predominantly Mexican Americans, half of whom speak Spanish. The curriculum for residents, which is required, begins with a month-long orientation to introduce family medicine residents to the community. The doctors spend nearly 30 hours on issues related to cultural competence, during which time they learn about traditional healers and community-oriented primary care and hold small-group discussions, readings, and self-reflective exercises. Throughout the year, issues related to cultural competence are integrated into the standard teaching curriculum and codified in a manual. Residents present clinical cases to faculty regularly, with particular emphasis on the sociocultural perspective. In addition, a yearly faculty development retreat helps integrate cultural competence into all of the teaching at White Memorial (Betancourt et al., 2002; Felt-Lisk and Kleinman, 2000).

Work in Interdisciplinary Teams

The *Quality Chasm* report (Institute of Medicine, 2001:83) envisions a future in which clinicians "understand the advantage of high levels of cooperation, coordination and standardization to guarantee excellence, continuity, and reliability. Cooperation in patient care is more important than professional prerogatives and roles. There is a focus on good communication among members of a team, using all the expertise and knowledge of team members, and where appropriate, sensibly extending roles to meet patients' needs." As discussed in Chapter 3, this level of cooperation and coordination across all the professions is not yet a reality. There is generally a great lack of understanding among the professions for what each profession does, its level of training and education, and its existing or potential competencies. The absence of a common language, differing philosophies, politics, and turf battles across the professions remain the norm.

This situation is exacerbated by the fact that in the vast majority of educational settings, health professionals are socialized in isolation, hierarchy is fostered, and individual responsibility and decision making are relied upon almost exclusively (Hall and Weaver, 2001). Health professions education occurs largely in an environment of separately housed professional schools and separate clinical arenas governed by powerful separate deans, directors, and department chairs. Professional schools also have their own separate faculty, school calendars, and different points of entry into the profession. Frequently, separate schedules prevent the development of new courses and innovative curriculum design (Holmes, 1999). A lack of appreciation of the actual or potential contributions of each of the health professions is reinforced by such settings, and more important, students learn little about the high levels of coordination and collaboration needed to provide quality care for Americans. There is a profound disconnect between current role-oriented, isolated academic preparation and practice environments that rely on teams or

wish to do so (Stumpf and Clark, 1999).

One key to fostering interdisciplinary practice is interdisciplinary education, whereby a group of students from the health-related occupations with different educational backgrounds learn and interact together during certain periods of their education in order to collaborate in providing health-related services (Holmes, 1999). Educating the professions together affords students the opportunity to develop the collaborative relationships essential for cross-fertilization among disciplines in the practice environment and supports respect among the disciplines as well (Hayward et al., 1996).

There are many examples of successful efforts to provide education in working in teams and in developing team-related skills in a variety of care settings (Hall and Weaver, 2001; Headrick et al., 1996; Lavin et al., 2001; McCallin, 2001; Zwarenstein, 1999). One example involves an interdisciplinary team of student nurses, physical therapists, occupational therapists, and patient care assistants who developed interventions around patient activity and mobility, resulting in reduced incidence of immobility-associated complications (Markey and Brown, 2002). In another example, teams of students in physical and occupational therapy, speech and language therapy, and exercise physiology worked over a semester to provide wellness and prevention interventions to the homeless and the chronically ill senior population (Hamel, 2001).

Although such successful examples exist (Murray et al., 2000), interdisciplinary education has yet to become the norm in health professions education. This is true despite efforts over the past 50 years on the part of foundations, private organizations, and government agencies, with enthusiasm waxing and waning, often in relationship to funding support. In 1995, fewer than 15 percent of U.S. nursing and medical schools had any interdisciplinary programs (Larson, 1995) despite the calls for this approach for decades from a variety of disciplines (American Association of Colleges of Nursing, 1995;

Health Resources and Services Administration, 1999; National League for Nursing Interdisciplinary Health Education Panel, 1998; Pharmacy Deans Task Force on Professionalism, 2000). Although some professions and programs have revised their mission statements and written learning objectives related to interdisciplinary teams, few have set benchmarks and standards that all students must attain before graduation (Stephenson et al., 2002).

One barrier is that differences persist around the roles of team members and interprofessional relationships and attitudes among students (Hall and Weaver, 2001). A recent study of health professions students revealed that medical residents were less inclined overall toward interdisciplinary teamwork, although residents in internal medicine or family practice and students of advanced practice nursing and masters-level social work were positively inclined (Leipzig et al., 2002). The researchers concluded that for physicians, exposure to interdisciplinary

teamwork and team decision making needs to occur earlier than residency training. Other studies have echoed the notion that early introduction to interdisciplinary education is key to success (Horak et al., 1998).

Some of the reluctance on the part of schools that educate health professionals to embark on interdisciplinary education is related to the limited research on the effect of such education on interdisciplinary practice and patient care (Zwarenstein, 1999). Some fear that professional identities, hierarchies, and power relationships may be diluted if the focus becomes interdisciplinary (Headrick et al., 1998b). Many questions about when, whom, and how to educate remain unanswered and are open to future research (Hall and Weaver, 2001), though preliminary studies show that problem-based learning is highly effective for training students in teams (Brickell and Cole, 1996). Box 4-2 provides selected examples of successful efforts in interdisciplinary education.

Box 4-2. Interdisciplinary Education: Selected Examples

Eastern North Carolina Interdisciplinary Rural Health Model began in 1993 with students in health education, medicine, nursing, nutrition, pharmacology, and social work who were recruited for rotations in a community health/migrant health clinic in rural North Carolina. Researchers evaluated the effort in 1998 and noted that the educational strategies and curriculum evolved with community input. A follow-up study showed that the program enhanced student learning, strengthened the infrastructure and commitment of the university for decentralized education, and led to the development of team-based care paths and changes in the attitudes of providers regarding interdisciplinary service learning (Hagar, 2001; Holmes, 1999; Lilley et al., 1998).

Funded by the John A. Hartford Foundation, the **Great Lakes Geriatric Interdisciplinary Team Training** project was a 3-year collaborative effort involving two large health systems and their academic partners in two cities: **University Hospitals Health System, Case Western Reserve University,** and **Benjamin Rose Institute** in Cleveland, and the **Henry Ford Health System** and **Wayne State University** in Detroit. The purpose of the effort was to develop, implement, and evaluate a new model of interdisciplinary team training for medical residents, nurse practitioner students, and social work students. Representatives from these institutions chose 22 diverse training sites that exhibited a commitment to allowing time for participation in the didactic portions of the

(Continued on page 81)

(Continued from page 80)

program, time and space for teams to meet and work together, and e-mail and Internet access for electronic communication and distance learning. Core learning teams from the three disciplines, practicing on-site clinicians, and others involved in patient care were trained in the theoretical foundation of learning teams, team tools and techniques, team skills needed to address common geriatric problems, and use of electronic communications. Team meetings were scheduled each week to discuss the progress of patients and consider others who might benefit from interdisciplinary team treatment, as well as quality improvement for systems and processes. As teams became more expert in their skills, outside facilitators assisted them in adopting a self-facilitation mode, with the role of team leader being rotated among the members. Team projects included the development of a protocol for monitoring the drug intake and outcomes of patients with dementia, a protocol on how to approach families dealing with end-of-life decisions, and a continuous improvement project aimed at identifying and treating elder abuse more effectively.

Source: Great Lakes Geriatric Interdisciplinary Team Training (GITT) (2002)

Employ Evidence-Based Practice

Given the constant changes in knowledge and management of health care systems, a major challenge for the educational process is to prepare students for lifelong learning. As explored in Chapter 2, the amount of knowledge that health professionals must acquire has grown immensely. Genomics, proteomics, neuroscience, epidemiology, and emerging infectious diseases, especially as they relate to bioterrorism, are just some of the recent additions to the expanding knowledge base needed to use new diagnostic and therapeutic agents for the 21st century.

Professionals in training cannot hope to provide competent care to patients over their career unless they have the ability to update their knowledge and skills. The formal curricula of health professional schools are dated almost as soon as students graduate. The traditional emphasis, especially in medicine, on teaching a core of knowledge focused largely on the basic mechanisms of disease and pathophysiological principles, with the expectation that students will memorize the hundreds of facts presented to them, is outdated in light of this ever-expanding knowledge base. William Stead, Vanderbilt University, noted at the summit:

The root of the problem stems from the design of our curricula...the curriculum places a premium on individual knowledge. And that individual knowledge is memorized, and it's applied with individual flair. That works in what [can be] referred to as medical care, or for an acute problem where we can actually fix it. It does not work in a case where the rate of development of knowledge exceeds what you can learn and retain. If you read two articles every night, you're 500 years behind at the end of the first year. That's if you remember those two articles. (Stead, 2002)

Many medical schools are making strides in shifting away from rote memorization and incorporating evidence-based practice as part of the curriculum (Grad et al., 2001) In a 1999 AAMC survey, however, more than a quarter of the graduates of the 88 percent of medical schools teaching skills related to evidence-based medicine reported feeling unprepared to interpret clinical data, research, literature reviews, and critiques (American Association of Medical Colleges, 1999a). A national survey of internal medicine Association residency programs found that 37 percent of those surveyed had a freestanding evidence-based practice curriculum, but fewer than half offered faculty development in this area or performed an evaluation of the course (Green, 2000).

As discussed in Chapter 3, the collection of evidence related to the contribution of nursing to care has been thwarted in part by a failure to gather relevant data at practice sites. This lack of data has impacted the diffusion of evidence-based practice into nursing curricula. Scattered educational experiences exist (French, 1999), but these are not the norm.

Most programs that grant doctor of pharmacy degrees require coursework in subjects related to skills needed for evidence-based practice. These include courses in statistics, drug information, literature evaluation, and research methodology, the latter being required least often. In a recent survey, however, only 12.9 percent of schools required an extensive project involving data collection, analysis, and write-up (Murphy et al., 1999). Like nursing, pharmacy is currently attempting to identify and disseminate evidence related to its profession (Etminan et al., 1998)

The teaching of evidence-based practice is thwarted in part by a lack of easily replicable teaching methods, and questions remain regarding how such courses are translated into practice (Norman and Shannon, 1998; Taylor et al., 2000). Work has been done on assessing the skills associated with learning about evidence-based practice and evaluating the ability of students to apply evidence in managing common clinical problems (Bradley and Humphris, 1999). Problem-based learning has also been shown to facilitate the development of critical appraisal skills, and collaboration between researchers and practitioners within and among disciplines has been found to enhance the diffusion of innovations in evidence-based practice (Lusardi et al., 2002; Rosswurm and Larrabee, 1999). The success of evidence-based instruction may also be related to the point at which it is offered. One study found that evidence-based instruction enhanced knowledge of epidemiology in undergraduate programs, but not necessarily at the residency level (Norman and Shannon, 1998). Box 4-3 presents selected examples of education in evidence-based practice.

Box 4-3. Education in Evidence-Based Practice:

Selected Examples

The **Center for Research and Evidence-Based Practice at the University of Rochester School of Nursing** holds an annual conference specifically devoted to teaching the foundation of evidence-based practice. After reviewing and critiquing the evidence, implications for best practice are discussed. Recent presentations include "How effective are insulin pumps for the regulation of blood glucose in children with Type 1 diabetes?" The center also co-partners with the **Strong Nursing Practice at the University of Rochester Medical Center** in the Advancing Research and Clinical Practice Through Close Collaboration (ARCC) model. Both contribute to support salaries for a team of doctorally prepared nurses whose role is to better integrate research and practice, and advance evidence-based practice within the community. The ARCC team assists nurses in searching for and appraising evidence to answer clinical questions, and in designing and receiving funding to conduct studies (Mazurek, 2002).

Faculty Development Institute Focused on Evidence-Based Practice in Allied Health was a national 4-day Faculty Development Institute program for dental hygiene,

(Continued on page 83)

(Continued from page 82)

occupational therapy, and physical therapy faculty that assessed evidence-based practice knowledge, skills, and teaching strategies in advance; taught skills onsite; and followed up with respect to curriculum integration. The program has shown a significant increase in evidence-based practice knowledge and strong self-reported preparation to integrate evidence-based practice into courses (Forrest and Miller, 2001).

Cook County Hospital and Rush Medical College, Chicago, Illinois, instituted an evidence-based medicine course for first-year internal medicine residents taught by senior faculty and chief residents, covering question formulation, literature searching, critical appraisal skills, and application of results to the patient. A comparison of these students with a control group found that the structured educational intervention over a 7-week period produced substantial and durable improvements in residents' cognitive and technical evidence-based practice skills (Smith et al., 2000).

Apply Quality Improvement

Current evidence for educational activities in quality improvement across the health professions is sparse. There is little available information on the extent to which students are educated in such skill areas as error reduction, process measurement and redesign, and monitoring of patient data (Headrick et al., 1998a; Henley, 2002; Mosher and Colton, 2001).

In medicine, scattered experiences in educating students or residents in quality improvement principles have been documented. Researchers recently tested a new quality improvement curriculum by comparing a group of internal medicine students who took the course with a control group who did not. The intervention group scored significantly higher scores on post-tests compared with the control group (Ogrinc et al., 2002). One course at the University of Illinois College of Medicine at Rockford had a quality improvement curriculum in which students performed a series of chart audits of diabetes and made improvement recommendations to clinic directors (Henley, 2002). In another study, resident involvement was deemed critical to the success of a quality improvement intervention that significantly decreased the use of unnecessary intravenous catheters (Parenti et al., 1994). Recent efforts by AAMC have articulated the learning objectives and educational strategies that should be used to integrate quality improvement into education (American Association of Medical Colleges, 2001).

In nursing, content on quality improvement is most commonly incorporated into lectures within management courses and rarely included in clinical courses. Moreover, most nursing education programs have not required students to implement quality improvement strategies in clinical areas through experiential learning strategies (Buerhaus and Norman, 2001).

A large barrier to education in this competency is the shortage of practitioners knowledgeable in practices of quality improvement who can understand and implement quality improvement innovations in their clinical settings. With regard to safety in particular, surveys have shown that there is a shortage of teachers and researchers who have a profound understanding of how safety is maintained and can pass on those insights and associated innovations (Croskerry et al., 2000; Institute of Medicine, 2000). Moreover, the shift from traditional classroom-based lectures to project-oriented learning that is required for quality improvement activities is a source of tension for some educators (Schillinger et al., 2000). Evaluation of quality improvement activities also remains an issue, with student satisfaction scores or other less rigorous measures being the norm (Baker et al., 1998; Gordon et al., 1996; Headrick et al., 1998a; Weeks et al., 2000). A recent study by Ogrinc et al. (2002) made some progress on this front by developing a more reliable method for evaluating a quality improvement course for medical residents.

Quality improvement is usually discussed in terms of teams improving processes or systems, but there is another aspect of quality improvement that is more narrowly focused on the individual clinician—continuous self-assessment. There is as yet no clear understanding of how health professionals are or should be educated to reflect on their own performance strengths and weaknesses in order to identify learning needs, conduct a review of their performance, and reinforce new skills or behaviors so they can improve their performance. Education that addresses the various dimensions of ensuring continuing competency past the initial preparation for practice therefore requires attention.

Box 4-4 describes selected examples of educational programs that have addressed quality improvement.

Box 4-4. Education in Quality Improvement: Selected Examples

At **Chippewa Valley Technical College,** Eau Claire, Wisconsin, nursing students participated in a health care organization's continuous quality improvement project targeting patient safety. Students were actively involved in chart review and became acutely aware of safety issues related to medication administration, order transcription and implementation, and documentation (Taylor, 2001).

As part of the **Undergraduate Medical Education for the 21st Century (UME-21)** project, the **University of Connecticut School of Medicine** developed and implemented a quality improvement curriculum. Seventy-seven second-year students working in groups of two to four conducted quality improvement projects on diabetes mellitus at 24 community-based primary care practices. They collected baseline data, implemented a results-specific intervention, and reassessed quality indicators 6 months later. The rate of documentation of foot and eye exams increased significantly from baseline to remeasurement, and the mean value for glycohemoglobin dropped at remeasurement (Gould et al., 2002).

A multiyear effort by the **Institute of Health Care Improvement** brought together interdisciplinary teams from numerous health care organizations to work on specific health issues, for example, reducing cesarean deliveries, improving outcomes and reducing costs in adult cardiac surgery, and improving asthma care for adults and children. In the case of asthma care, 9 of 12 interdisciplinary teams from 12 medical centers had achieved sizeable reductions in hospital and emergency room visits within 15 months (Headrick et al., 1998b).

Utilize Informatics

Without a basic education in informatics, health professionals are limited in their ability to make effective use of communication and information technology in their practice. Yet without appropriate input from health professionals skilled in informatics, it may be impossible to implement a clinical computing infrastructure that meets the needs of clinicians and patients. Educating health professionals in informatics should enable many important capabilities, including appropriate interaction with clinical information systems for making decisions and mitigating error, use of the Internet to inform themselves and their patients, and facility in using e-mail to communicate and coordinate with their team members and patients.

Though many studies focus on the use of computers in the delivery of educational content, very few studies document how students or professionals in practice are educated to use information technology in support of patient care. Many institutions are now offering degrees (masters and doctorate), fellowships, certificates, and short courses in this area, some through remote learning; the website of the American Medical Informatics Association (2002) lists over 50 such programs. However, these are usually special degrees and optional courses not required of the professions.

According to findings from a 1999 AAMC medical school graduation questionnaire, about 86 percent of respondents felt comfortable using the Web to locate and acquire information, and nearly three-quarters felt confident about using a computer-based clinical record-keeping program for both finding and recording patient-specific information (American Association of Medical Colleges, 1999b). During 2000–2001, 46 percent of medical schools required their students to own or rent personal computers (Barzansky and Etzel, 2001). AAMC, through the Medical School Objectives Project, recently identified core informatics competencies in medicine (American Association of Medical Colleges, 1999b).

Probably as a result of resource constraints in the settings in which they are educated, nursing and allied health professionals have embraced informatics on a more limited scale as compared with their medical counterparts (Gassert, 1998; Hovenga, 2000; McDaniel et al., 1998). Community colleges, where the majority of registered nurses are trained, do not provide access to information technology to the same extent as academic medical centers. A 1998 survey of accredited diploma, associates, bachelors, and masters nursing programs revealed that a majority of schools lacked a coordinated plan for technology implementation and were underfinanced for technology and related personnel; fewer than one-third of the schools addressed nursing informatics in the curriculum (Carty and Rosenfeld, 1998).

Issues around competencies associated with the use of informatics and whether they are discipline-specific or broad-based hinder progress on widespread education in this area (Masys et al., 2000). One recent effort to address discipline-specific competencies has been the International Medical Informatics Association recommendations regarding courses by profession, by type of specialization in health, and by stage of career progression (e.g., bachelors, masters). These recommendations address educational programs in medicine, nursing, health care management, dentistry, pharmacology, public health, health record administration, and informatics/computer science, as well as dedicated health informatics programs (American Medical Informatics Association, 2002). Another example is the multitiered set of technology competencies specifically designed for occupational therapy practitioners authored by the American Occupational Therapy Association Technology Special Interest Section (Hammel and Angelo, 1996).

A number of issues help explain the current barriers to integrating informatics into health professions curriculum: the lack of a clear understanding of informatics as a discipline, limited support for informatics education among administrators and faculty, the overcrowded nature of existing curricula, inadequate time for faculty to develop associated skills (Jerant, 1999), and the lack of quick and easy access to local informatics experts (Cartwright et al., 2002). The difficulty in conceptualizing informatics education is often exacerbated by a "tendency to conflate education in informatics with the use of computers to deliver education" (Buckeridge and Goel, 2002:4). Interacting with computing resources in the educational process is not the same as applying informatics to patient care. Box 4-5 describes some examples of successful efforts to provide education on the use of informatics.

Box 4-5. Education in Informatics: Selected Examples

The Educational Services Department, New York University Medical Center, introduced a multidisciplinary informatics curriculum including a menu of offerings that can be adapted to meet the varying skills, needs, and schedules of clinicians; basic scientists; residents; and medical, nursing, and allied health students. Offerings include workshops in basic computer skills, the identification of information resources, the structure of information, the development of search strategies in support of evidence-based practice, the identification of qualitative journal literature, and critical appraisal of the literature (Faraino, 1998).

Florida State University College of Medicine, Tallahassee, Florida, is spending 6.6 percent of its annual budget on information technology. To ensure that students have access to the latest hardware and software, they are provided fully loaded laptops and personal digital assistants (PDAs). The school plans to store all teaching cases in electronic medical records. Training in skills related to computer and information mastery to advanced levels is also provided. Informatics skills are integrated into every teaching case in the doctoring course for years one and two, and tested in objective structured clinical examinations along with clinical skills thereafter (Scherger, 2002).

The Center for Advanced Technology in Surgery, Stanford University, Palo Alto, California, anticipates over the next 10 years selecting, training, credentialing, remediating, and recredentialing physicians and surgeons using simulation, virtual reality, and Web-based electronic learning. The center anticipates that future physicians will be able to rehearse an operation on a projectable palpable hologram derived from patient-specific data, and deliver the dataset of that operation with robotic assistance the next day. A simulator-based curriculum developed by Stanford in conjunction with the Veterans Affairs Palo Alto Health Care System has been built upon by other institutions, including Harvard Medical School (Gorman et al., 2000; Robeznieks, 2002).

A Vision of the Future Health Professions Student

The five competencies described in this chapter define the environment that leaders in health professions education, such as those who attended the Health Professions Education Summit, must address. These competencies can enable both students and practicing professionals to better meet the needs of patients. Box 4-6 presents a scenario depicting an educational experience as it could be if these competencies were incorporated into the curriculum of the health professions.

Box 4-6. A Vision of Health Professions Education for the Future

Monica Clarke, Justin Howell, and María Gonzalez are fellow health sciences students at the University of Brobdingnag Health Sciences Center. Monica is a medical student, Justin is a nursing student, and María is a pharmacy student. They serve as an integrated health team, and have been assigned for the duration of their 10-week rotation to see internal medicine cases at the university hospital, with follow-up in a community health facility. The university employs interdisciplinary teams throughout the health sciences center in both teaching and health care delivery contexts. Accordingly, a faculty internist, assisted by an acute care nurse practitioner and a pharmacist, leads the students' team.

At the beginning of their shift at the hospital, the team admits Mr. Ruiz to their service. Mr. Ruiz, a 55-year-old construction worker, presented to the hospital emergency department (ED) yesterday with an episode of severe chest pain. Rapid evaluation in the ED revealed that he was experiencing an acute myocardial infarction, and he was rushed to the catheterization laboratory, where a blocked coronary artery was opened with angioplasty. He rested comfortably overnight in the cardiology care unit, and was transferred to the internal medicine team for further management and follow-up.

To quickly familiarize themselves with Mr. Ruiz's case, the students consult their handheld computers, which provide full access to Mr. Ruiz's current hospital chart, as well as notes from his previous visits to a community health facility. Information about his previous examinations, medication profiles, radiology reports, and electrocardiograms are all available electronically. Consulting Mr. Ruiz's ED notes, the team members note that Mr. Ruiz had been seen at the community health facility 2 years ago and had been noted as having mildly elevated blood pressure, but had not returned to the clinic since.

Together, the students, by referring to Mr. Ruiz's electronic record and interviewing him, confirm and complete his full medical history, including previous medications, issues raised and recorded by the nursing staff since he was admitted, and family history. The information is stored using an electronic template on the health system's server, where it will be easily accessible for future use by any of Mr. Ruiz's health care team. The interview reveals that Mr. Ruiz takes several over-the-counter analgesics and an herbal medicine. He smokes two packs of cigarettes daily. There are several cases of noninsulin diabetes in his immediate family. Until the episode of chest pain yesterday that prompted his trip to the ED, he was unaware of any other medical problems. During his interview, he expresses his concern about both the cost of his hospitalization and the implications of his heart attack for his employment.

(Continued on page 88)

(Continued from page 87)

Monica and Justin perform a physical examination, with guidance from their faculty. His vital signs are stable, and his catheterization wound site is healing well, although he is overweight. After discussion among themselves and their faculty, the students decide to order a routine follow-up EKG and some blood tests. The EKG reveals no evidence of acute ischemia or other abnormalities. At the same time, the team's handheld devices flash to note that the laboratory results reveal elevated cholesterol, elevated blood glucose, and mild renal dysfunction, although the level of his cardiac enzymes has decreased since his admission, indicating improved blood flow to his heart after the angioplasty procedure.

The students compile a problem list for Mr. Ruiz. He has coronary artery disease, diabetes, high cholesterol, and mild renal disease. He has recently suffered an acute myocardial infarction, abuses tobacco, and is well above his optimal weight. He also has concerns about the cost of his medical care, as well as his ability to continue working. The students design an integrated plan that addresses current problems and seeks to prevent further injury and progression of these problems.

Monica researches appropriate diagnostics and therapy for Mr. Ruiz's coronary artery disease, diabetes, high cholesterol, and renal disease. She recruits assistance from the cardiology team regarding further cardiac testing, from the cardiac rehabilitation team to design an exercise program for Mr. Ruiz to assist in his recovery and eventual return to work, and from the diabetic team to advise on control of his disease and its complications.

Justin designs a health behavior change plan, drawing on the resources of the smoking cessation psychologist, the diabetic educator, and the dietician to begin the process of educating Mr. Ruiz about his medical and lifestyle issues, and then designing a program to help him manage his conditions. Justin also contacts a social worker to review Mr. Ruiz's health insurance plan to ensure that he is taking advantage of all financial resources available to him.

Maria investigates Mr. Ruiz's previous medication history, including his herbal medicine, to determine whether any potential interactions exist between them and the medicines that Mr. Ruiz will now require to manage his conditions. She works to tailor his medication regime to maximize benefit while minimizing cost, complexity, and side effects.

As the students perform their tasks, they validate their work using the clinical decision support capability available on the health system's computer network. The decision support system offers possible treatment options derived from current research, clinical guidelines, and clinical expert opinion. The system also offers medical databases, such as MEDLINE, that enable the students to research the latest medical, nursing, and pharmacy treatments available. The students consider Mr. Ruiz's preferences and individual conditions, and then select the most appropriate therapy. When Monica attempts to prescribe two medicines with a potentially serious interaction, her handheld computer flashes a warning. Working together, she and Maria propose a more suitable alternative.

At the completion of their work, and with approval from their faculty members, they present their treatment plan to Mr. Ruiz. He expresses interest in the plan, and makes some suggestions about ways to integrate the changes into his life. He spends the rest of his hospital stay learning about his conditions and treatments, both from his team and from an informational website accessible on his bedside computer. He is taught to monitor his

(Continued on page 89)

(Continued from page 88)

own blood pressure and given a log to record his blood pressure and his nutritional, drug, and herbal intake, as well as his exercise activities and symptoms. He is discharged to follow-up in 2 weeks at the community health facility. During the interim, he has a question regarding one of his medicines, and he calls the clinic, where his question is answered by one of the nurse practitioners on duty.

Two weeks later, Mr. Ruiz arrives at the community health facility for follow-up with his log in hand and is seen by the same student team. They evaluate Mr. Ruiz's progress, note his interim medication question, and fine-tune his follow-up plan based on the results of an examination and new laboratory tests, as well as on input from Mr. Ruiz himself. His electronic medical record is updated with the new information, and he is automatically registered in both coronary artery disease and diabetes databases, which serve to remind his health team of periodic tests and exams that are indicated. The databases are reviewed periodically by the health system to ensure that his care and outcomes are in accordance with best practices. At the end of their rotation, the students download the treatment plan for Mr. Ruiz, as well as those of the other patients for whom they cared, and review them with their faculty. Successes and missed opportunities are discussed, and methods for improvement are highlighted.

Outcome-Based Education

Identification of general competencies represents an articulation of what health professionals should know and be able to do. In the previous chapter, the committee defined five competencies that it deems critical for all clinicians to possess, with the understanding that the way in which these competencies are integrated into educational programs will be discipline-specific. In this chapter, the committee has explored the extent to which such competencies are addressed in educational curricula.

The identification of competencies is not an isolated activity—identifying competencies is just the first of many steps in ensuring that students are prepared to deliver quality health care. Once competencies have been established, the knowledge, skills, and attitudes underpinning each competency need to be clearly articulated in writing and related measures developed. Assessment tools must then be matched to each competency to evaluate outcomes—the results providing evidence that goals and objectives have been accomplished (Carraccio et al., 2002; Calhoun, 2002). This

articulation of what students should be able to do and of education based on related objectives is often referred to as *competency-based* or *outcome-based education.*

Epstein and Hundert (2002) note that the outcomes of assessment serve many needs for learners, academic institutions, and the public, including the following:

- Learner—fosters learning, inspires confidence, and enhances the ability to self-monitor.

- Curriculum—drives change, certifies achievement of curricular goals, and creates coherence.

- Academic institutions—drives self-assessment, expresses values, serves to develop faculty, and provides data for educational research.

- Public—certifies competence of graduates, and offers comparative data on the quality of educational programs.

Hendricson and Cohen (2001) outline three questions that educational institutions must answer to develop competency-based health professions education:

- What knowledge, skills, and professional/ personal values should the student possess at the time of graduation so he or she will be ready for the next level of training (e.g., a postgraduate year one) or be prepared to serve as an independently functioning entry-level general practitioner?

- What learning experiences will enable students to acquire these competencies?

- What proof, or evidence, is needed to establish for faculty that a student has attained competency?

Hendricson and Cohen describe a competency-based curriculum as ideally having three features: (1) top-down planning based on analysis of the health care needs of patients, (2) a readiness-based model in which students advance through the curriculum at different rates based on their individual capabilities, and (3) a horizontal curriculum structure in which students progress through competency modules hierarchically sequenced by level of difficulty.

Scattered clinical education institutions have restructured their curricula and student learning methods using a competency-based approach (DeWald and McCann, 1999). However, little attention has been devoted to defining the standards for such competencies; determining how to attain them; or evaluating competence, particularly with respect to professionalism and humanism. Each of these areas remains a large challenge (Carraccio et al., 2002).

A major impediment to moving towards competency-based education is making additions to existing overcrowded curricula. Some institutions have integrated competencies as "themes" into existing coursework rather than instituting new courses. Examples of themes that are woven into the entire education experience include evidence-based practice, ethics, and AIDS (Dartmouth Medical School, 1998; Harvard Medical School, 2000). At the same time, the environment for health professions education is changing with respect

to the use of computers and new educational approaches, such as problem based learning—which in combination may allow the same amount of content to be conveyed more efficiently and effectively. One 3-year study of a new curriculum that integrated computer-based activities and problem-based learning found that students could identify and retrieve information more rapidly and were more self-reliant in solving problems, therefore making fewer time demands of faculty and tutors. This new curriculum also resulted in reducing laboratory time from the national norm of 141 hours to 93 hours (Levine et al., 1999).

Educational reformers posit that by supporting students in directing their own learning and providing the tools they need to access, analyze, and apply information, education will be transformed. Distance learning technology, standardized patients, and clinical skills-testing techniques also hold the potential for revolutionizing health professions education, offering students the opportunity to customize their learning and to progress at their own pace and at geographic locations that meet their educational needs. Of course, such an approach would need to be closely monitored by faculty and validated through testing.

Colleen Conway-Welch, Vanderbilt University, commented at the summit on the need to focus more on students:

> Wouldn't it be interesting if we also thought that the student was the center of the educational system? And perhaps, if the focus moved to the patient and the student, that might reinforce this whole idea that they are both highly valued. And the students then may start asking some of the tougher questions because they themselves feel that they have been valued in the process and can transfer some of those learnings over to the patient. Perhaps we could accelerate this change (Conway-Welch, 2002).

Conclusion

The committee concludes with the following observations on the current state of educational preparation in the five competencies:

- **The extent to which health professionals are prepared to achieve the five competencies necessary for optimum patient-centered care requires more standardization across and within the professions.**

- **The core set of competencies needs to be integrated more thoroughly into a cohesive educational experience and to be offered using interactive methods.**

- **Evaluation of the effects of health professions education requires increased attention. Few investigators study whether curricula, courses, or teaching methods are having the desired impact on learners and their practice or on the delivery of health care to the American public. When evaluations are done, they often do not have the types of designs necessary to provide an adequate understanding of those effects.**

References

Great Lakes Geriatric Interdisciplinary Team Training (GITT). Online. Available at http://gitt.cwru.edu/ [accessed Sept., 2002].

Allen, C.E. 2000. Public health nursing vital. *Nations Health* 30 (5):3.

American Association of Colleges of Nursing. 1995. *Interdisciplinary Education and Practice.* California: AACN.

———. 2002. "Recommended Competencies and Curricular Guidelines for End-of-Life Nursing Care." Online. Available at http://www.aacn.nche.edu/publications/deathfin.htm [accessed Sept., 2002].

American Association of Colleges of Pharmacy

Commission to Implement Change in Pharmaceutical Education. 1993. What is the mission of pharmacy education. *American Journal of Pharmacy Education* 57:374-76.

American Association of Medical Colleges. 1999a. *Evidence Based Medicine Instruction* . Vol 2, No.3 edition Washington, DC: AAMC.

———. 1999b. *Keeping Up with Technology and the Changing Role of Medicine* . Vol 2 No.2 edition Washington, DC: AAMC.

American Association of Medical Colleges. 2000. *Report III: Communication in Medicine. Medical School Objectives Project.* Washington, DC: Assoication of American Medical Colleges.

American Association of Medical Colleges. 2001. *Report V - Contemporary Issues in Medicine: Quality of Care.* Washington, DC: Association of American Medical Colleges.

American Medical Informatics Association. 2002. "AMIA Web site." Online. Available at www.amia.org [accessed Feb. 15, 2002].

American Pharmacuetical Association. 2002. "Principles of Practice for Pharmaceutical Care." Online. Available at http://www.aphanet.org/pharmcare/prinprac.html [accessed 2002].

Baker, G.R., S. Gelmon, L. Headrick, M. Knapp, L. Norman, D. Quinn, and D. Neuhauser. 1998. Collaborating for improvement in health professions education. *Quality Management in Health Care* 6 (2):1-11.

Barzansky, B., and S.I. Etzel. 2001. Educational programs in U.S. medical schools, 2000-2001. *Journal of the American Medical Association* 286 (9):1049-55.

Beardsley, R.S. 2001. Communication skills development in colleges of pharmacy. *American Journal of Pharmaceutical Education* 65 (4)

Beisecker, A.E., R.A. Murden, W.P. Moore, D. Graham, and L. Nelmig. 1996. Attitudes of medical students and primary care physicians regarding input of older and younger patients in medical decisions. *Medical Care* 34 (2):126-37.

Betancourt, J.R., A. R. Green, and J. E.Carrillo. 2002. *Cultural Competence in Health Care: Emerging Frameworks and Practical Approaches.*The Commonwealth Fund.

Bloom, S.W. 1989. The medical school as a social organization: The sources of resistance to change. *Medical Education* 23 (3):228-41.

Bradley, P., and G. Humphris. 1999. Assessing the ability of medical students to apply evidence in practice: The potential of the OSCE. *Medical Education* 33 (11):815-17.

Branch, W.T., Jr. 2000. Supporting the moral development of medical students. *Journal of General Internal Medicine* 15 (7):503-8.

Branch, W.T., Jr. MD, D. Kern, P. Haidet, P. Weissmann, C.F. Gracey, G. Mitchell, and T. Inui. 2001. The patient-physician relationship. Teaching the human dimensions of care in clinical settings. *Journal of American Medical Association* 286 (9):1067-74.

Brickell, J.M., and C.M. Cole. 1996. Using a problem-based learning format to teach CLS students interdisciplinary health care practice. *Clinical Laboratory Science* 9 (1):48-54.

Buckeridge, D.L. and V. Goel. 2002. Medical informatics in an undergraduate curriuclum: An qualitative study. *Bio Medical Central Medical Informatics and Decision Making* 2 (6):1-5.

Buerhaus, P.I., and L. Norman. 2001. Its time to require theory and methods of quality improvement in basic and graduate nursing education. *Nursing Outlook* 49 (2):67-69.

Calhoun, J.G., P.L. Davidson, M.E. Sinioris, E.T. Vincent, and J.R. Griffith. 2002. Toward an understanding of competency identification and assessment in health care management. *Qual Manag Health Care* 11(1):14-38.

Carraccio, C., S.D. Wolfsthal, R. Englander, K. Ferentz, and C. Martin. 2002. Shifting paradigms: From flexner to competencies. *Academic Medicine* 77 (5):361-67.

Cartwright, C.A., N. Korsen, and L.E. Urbach. 2002. Teaching the teachers: Helping faculty in a family practice residency improve their informatics skills. *Academic Medicine* 77 (5):385-91.

Carty, B., and P. Rosenfeld. 1998. From computer technology to information technology. Findings from a national study of nursing education. *Computer Nursing* 16 (5):259-65.

Center for the Advancement of Pharmaceutical Education [CAPE] Advisory Panel on

Educational Outcomes. 1998. "Educational Outcomes." Online. Available at http://www. aacp.org/Docs/MainNavigation/ Resources/3933_edoutcom.doc? DocTypeID=4&TrackID=&VID=1&CID=410& DID=366 [accessed Dec. 10, 2002].

Chisholm, M.A., and W.E. Wade. 1999. Factors influencing students attitudes toward pharmaceutical care. *Am J Health Syst Pharm* 56 (22):2330-2335.

Collins, T., K. Goldenberg, A. Ring, K. Nelson, and J. Konen. 1991. The Association of Teachers of Preventive Medicines recommendations for postgraduate education in prevention. *Academic Medicine* 66 (6):317-20.

Conway-Welch, C. 2002. ""Crossing the Quality Chasm: Next Steps for Health Professions Education"; Panel Discussion." Online. Available at http://www.kaisernetwork.org/ health_cast/hcast_index.cfm? display=detail&hc=601 [accessed Nov. 12, 2002].

Croskerry, P., R.L. Wears, and L.S. Binder. 2000. Setting the educational agenda and curriculum for error prevention in emergency medicine. [Review] [40 refs]. *Academic Emergency Medicine* 7 (11):1194-2000.

Dartmouth Medical School. 1998. "Welcome to the integrated primary care clerkship--IPCC." Online. Available at http://cobweb.dartmouth. edu/~biomed/IPCC/ [accessed 2002].

DeWald, J.P., and A.L. McCann. 1999. Developing a competency-based curriculum for a dental hygiene program. *Journal of Dental Education* 63 (11):793-804.

Epstein, R.M., and E.M. Hundert. 2002. Defining and assessing professional competence. *Journal of the American Medical Association* 287 (2):226-35.

Etminan, M., J.M. Wright, and B.C. Carleton. 1998. Evidence-based pharmacotherapy: Review of basic concepts and applications in clinical practice. *Annals of Pharmacotherapy* 32 (11):1193-2000.

Eyler, J.S., D.E. Giles, Jr. , C.M. Stenson, and C. J. Gray. 2001. *At A Glance: What We Know about The Effects of Service-Learning on College Students, Faculty, Institutions and Communities, 1993- 2000: Third Edition.*Corporation for

National Service Learn and Serve America National Service Learning Clearinghouse.

Faraino, R.L. 1998. Teaching medical informatics a la carte: A curriculum for the professional palate. *Medical Reference Services Quarterly* 17 (2):69-77.

Felt-Lisk, S., and L. Kleinman. 2000. *Effective Clinical Practice in Managed Care, Findings From Ten Case Studies*. Boston, MA: The Commonwealth Fund.

Flores, G., D. Gee, and B. Kastner. 2000. The teaching of cultural issues in U.S. and Canadian medical schools. *Academic Medicine* 75 (5):451-55.

Forrest, J.L., and S.A. Miller. 2001. Integrating evidence-based decision making into allied health curricula. *Journal of Allied Health* 30 (4):215-22.

French, P. 1999. The development of evidence-based nursing. *Journal of Advanced Medicine* 29 (1):72-78.

Garr, D.R., D.T. Lackland, and D.B. Wilson. 2000. Prevention education and evaluation in U.S. medical schools: A status report. *Academic Medicine* 75 (7):14S-21.

Gassert, C.A. 1998. The challenge of meeting patients needs with a national nursing informatics agenda. *Journal of the American Medical Informatics Association* 5 (3):263-68.

Gerteis, M., S. Edgman-Levitan, J. Daley, and T. Delbanco, editors. 1993. *Through the Patient Eyes*. Vol. San Francisco, CA: Josey-Bass.

Gordon, P.R., L. Carlson, A. Chessman, M.L. Kundrat, P.S. Morahan, and L.A. Headrick. 1996. A multisite collaborative for the development of interdisciplinary education in continuous improvement for health professions students. *Academic Medicine* 71 (9):973-78.

Gorman, P.J.M., A.H.M. Meier, C. Rawn, and T.M. M. Krummel. 2000. The future of medical education is no longer blood and guts, it is bits and bytes. *American Journal of Surgery* 180 (5):353-56.

Gould, B.E., M.R. Grey, C.G. Huntington, C. Gruman, J.H. Rosen, E. Storey, L. Abrahamson, A.M. Conaty, L. Curry, M. Ferreira, K.L. Harrington, D. Paturzo, and T.J. Van Hoof. 2002. Improving patient care outcomes by teaching quality improvement to medical students in community-based practices. *Academic Medicine* 77 (10):1011-18.

Grad, R., A.C. Macaulay, and M. Warner. 2001. Teaching evidence-based medical care: Description and evaluation. *Family Medicine* 33 (8):602-6.

Green, M.L. 2000. Evidence-based medicine training in internal medicine residency programs a national survey. *Journal of General Internal Medicine* 15 (2):129-33.

Hagar, M. 2001. *Enhancing Interactions Between Nursing and Medicine*. Chicago: Josiah Macy Jr. Foundation.

Hall, P., and L. Weaver. 2001. Interdisciplinary education and teamwork: A long and winding road. *Medical Education* 35 (9):867-75.

Halpern, R., M.Y. Lee, P.R. Boulter, and R.R. Phillips. 2001. A synthesis of nine major reports on physicians competencies for the emerging practice environment. *Academic Medicine* 76 (6):606-15.

Hamel, P.C. 2001. Interdisciplinary perspectives, service learning, and advocacy: A nontraditional approach to geriatric rehabilitation. *Topics in Geriatric Rehabilitation* 17 (1):53-70.

Hammel, J. and J. Angelo. 1996. Technology competencies for occupational therapy practitioners. *Assistive Technology* 8 (1):34-42.

Hamner, J., and B. Wilder. 2001. A new curriculum for a new millennium. *Nursing Outlook* 49 (3):127-31.

Harvard Medical School. 2000. "Themes Harvard Medical School." Online. Available at http://www.hms.harvard.edu/oed/themes2/ [accessed 2002].

Hayward, K.S., L.T. Powell, and J. McRoberts. 1996. Changes in student perceptions of interdisciplinary practice in the rural setting. *Journal of Allied Health* 25 (4):315-27.

Headrick, L.A., M. Knapp, D. Neuhauser, S. Gelmon, L. Norman, D. Quinn, and R. Baker. 1996. Working from upstream to improve health care: The IHI interdisciplinary professional education collaborative. *Joint Commission Journal on Quality Improvement* 22 (3):149-64.

Headrick, L.A., A. Richardson, and G.P. Priebe.

1998a. Continuous improvement learning for residents. *Pediatrics* 101 (4 Pt 2):768-73; discussion 773-774.

Headrick, L.A., P.M. Wilcock, and P.B. Batalden. 1998b. Continuing medical education: Interprofessional working and continuing medical education. *British Medical Journal* 316 (7133):771-74.

Health Resources and Services Administration. 1999. *Building the Future of Allied Health: Report of the Implementation Task Force of the National Commission on Allied Health.* Rockville, MD: Health Resources and Services Administration.

Heller, B.R., M.T. Oros, and J. Durney-Crowley. 2000. The future of nursing education. Ten trends to watch. *Nursing Health Care Perspectives* 21 (1):9-13.

Henbest, R.J., and M. Stewart. 1990. Patient-centredness in the consultation. 2: Does it really make a difference? *Family Practice* 7 (1):28-33.

Hendricson, W.D., and P.A. Cohen. 2001. Oral health care in the 21st century: Implications for dental and medical education. *Academic Medicine* 76 (12):1181-206.

Henley, E. 2002. A quality improvement curriculum for medical students. *Joint Commission Journal on Quality Improvement* 28 (1):42-48.

Holmes, D.E., and M. Osterweis. 1999. *Catalysts in Interdisciplinary Education.* Washington, DC: Association of Academic Health Centers.

Horak, B.J., K.C. O'Leary, and L. Carlson. 1998. Preparing health care professionals for quality improvement: The George Washington University/George Mason University experience. *Quality Management in Health Care* 6 (2):21-30.

Hovenga, E.J. 2000. Global health informatics education. *Studies in Health Technology & Informatics* 57:3-14.

Institute of Medicine. 1988. *The Future of Public Health.* Washington, DC: National Academy Press.

————. 1995. *Dental Education at a Crossroads.* Vol. Committee on the Future of Dental Education and Marilyn J. Field, eds.

Washington, DC: National Academy Press.

————. 2000. *To Err Is Human: Building a Safer Health System.* Linda T. Kohn, Janet M. Corrigan, and Molla S. Donaldson, eds. Washington, DC: National Academy Press.

————. 2001. *Improving Palliative Care for Cancer.* Washington, DC: National Academy Press.

————. 2002a. *Unequal Treatment: Confronting Racial and Ethnic Disparities in Health Care.* Washington, DC: National Academy Press.

————. 2002b. *When Children Die: Improving Palliative and End-of-Life Care for Children and Their Families.* Washington, DC: National Academy Press.

Institute of Medicine, H.P.E.S. 2001. Online [accessed 2002].

Jerant, A.F. 1999. Training residents in medical informatics. *Family Medicine* 31 (7):465-72.

Langewitz, W.A., P. Eich, A. Kiss, and B. Wossmer. 1998. Improving communication skills--a randomized controlled behaviorally oriented intervention study for residents in internal medicine. *Psychosomatic Medicine* 60 (3):268-76.

Larson, E.L. 1995. New rules for the game: Interdisciplinary education for health professionals. *Nursing Outlook* 43 (4):180-185.

Lavin, M.A., I. Ruebling, R. Banks, L. Block, M. Counte, G. Furman, P. Miller, C. Reese, V. Viehmann, and J. Holt. 2001. Interdisciplinary health professional education: A historical review. *Advances in Health Sciences Education* 6 (1):25-47.

Leipzig, R.M., K. Hyer, K. Ek, S. Wallenstein, M.L. Vezina, S. Fairchild, C.K. Cassel, and J.L. Howe. 2002. Attitudes Toward Working on Interdisciplinary Healthcare Teams: a Comparison by Discipline. *Journal of the American Geriatrics Society* 50 (6):1141-8.

Levine, M.G., J. Stempak, G. Conyers, and J.A. Walters. 1999. Implementing and integrating computer-based activities into a problem-based gross anatomy curriculum. *Clinical Anatomy* 12 (3):191-98.

Lewin, S.A., Z.C. Skea, V. Entwistle, M. Zwarenstein, and J. Dick. 2001. Interventions for providers to promote a patient-centred approach in clinical consultations (Cochrane Review). *Cochrane Database System Review* 4:CD003267.

Lilley, S.H., M. Clay, A. Greer, J. Harris, and H.D. Cummings. 1998. Interdisciplinary rural health training for health professional students: Strategies for curriculum design. *Journal of Allied Health* 27 (4):208-12.

Lipkin, M. 1996. Patient education and counseling in the context of modern patient-physician-family communication. [Review] [19 refs]. *Patient Education & Counseling* 27 (1):5-11.

Lusardi, M.M., P.K. Levangie, and B.D. Fein. 2002. A problem-based learning approach to facilitate evidence-based practice in entry-level health professional education. *Journal of Prosthetics & Orthotics June* 14 (2):40-50.

Maguire, P., K. Booth, C. Elliott, and B. Jones. 1996. Helping health professionals involved in cancer care acquire key interviewing skills--the impact of workshops. *European Journal of Cancer* 32A (9):1486-89.

Malloch, K., D. Sluyter, and N. Moore. 2000. Relationship-centered care: Achieving true value in healthcare. *Journal Nursing Administration* 30 (7-8):379-85.

Markey, D.W., and R.J. Brown. 2002. An Interdisciplinary Approach to Addressing Patient Activity and Mobility in the Medical-Surgical Patient. *Journal of Nursing Care Quality* 16 (4):1-12.

Marvel, M.K., R.M. Epstein, K. Flowers, and H.B. Beckman. 1999. Soliciting the patients agenda: Have we improved? *Journal of the American Medical Association* 281 (3):283-87.

Masys, D.R., P.F. Brennan, J.G. Ozbolt, M. Corn, and E.H. Shortliffe. 2000. Are medical informatics and nursing informatics distinct disciplines? The 1999 ACMI debate. *Journal of American Medical Information Association* 7 (3):304-12.

Mazurek, B. 2002. Strategies for overcoming barriers in implementing evidence-based practice. *Periatric Nursing* 28 (2):159-61.

McCallin, A. 2001. Interdisciplinary practice - a matter of teamwork: An integrated literature review. *Journal of Clinical Nursing* 10 (4):419-28.

McDaniel, A.M., C. Matlin, P.R. Elmer, K. Paul, and G. Monastiere. 1998. Computer use in staff development: A national survey. *Journal for Nurses in Staff Development* 14 (3):117-26.

Mead, N., and P. Bower. 2000. Patient-centredness: A conceptual framework and review of the empirical literature. *Social Science Medicine* 51 (7):1087-110.

Milio, N. 2002. A new leadership role for nursing in a globalized world. *Topics in Advanced Practice Nursing EJournal* 2 (1)

Mosher, S.A., and D. Colton. 2001. Quality improvement in the curriculum: A survey of AUPHA programs. *Journal of Health Administration Education* 19 (2):203-20.

Murawski, M., D. Murawski, and Wilson. 1999. Service-learning and pharmaceutical education: An exploratory survey. *American Journal of Pharmacy Education* 63 (1)

Murphy, J.E., L.S. Peralta, and D.M. Kirking . 1999. Research experiences and research-related coursework in the education of doctors of pharmacy. *Pharmacotherapy* 19 (2):213-20.

Murray, E., L. Gruppen, P. Catton, R. Hays, and J.O. Woolliscroft. 2000. The accountability of clinical education: Its definition and assessment. *Medical Education* 34 (10):871-79.

National League for Nursing Interdisciplinary Health Education Panel. 1998. Building community: Developing skills for interprofessional health profession education and relationship-centered care. *Nursing and Health Care Perspectives* 19:87-90.

Norman, G.R., and S.I. Shannon. 1998. Effectiveness of instruction in critical appraisal (evidence-based medicine) skills: a critical appraisal. *Canadian Medical Association Journal* 158 (2):177-81.

Novack, D.H., R.M. Epstein, and R.H. Paulsen. 1999. Toward creating physician-healers: fostering medical students self-awareness, personal growth, and well-being. [Review] [51 refs]. *Academic Medicine* 74 (5):516-50.

Ogrinc G., Headrick L.A., Morrison L.J., and Foster T. 2002. Teaching and Assessing Resident Competence in Practice-based Learning and Improvement A Non-randomized, Controlled Trial. *8th International Scientific Symposium on Improving Quality and Value in Health Care.*

ONeil, E. H. and the Pew Health Professions Commission. 1998. *Recreating health professional practice for a new century - The fourth report of the PEW health professions Commission.* San Francisco, CA: Pew Health Professions Commission.

Parenti, C.M., F.A. Lederle, C.L. Impola, and L.R. Peterson. 1994. Reduction of unnecessary intravenous catheter use. Internal medicine house staff participate in a successful quality improvement project. *Archives of Medicine* 154 (16):1829-32.

Peterson, C.A. 2001. Nursing shortage: Not a simple problem - no easy answers. *Online Journal of Issues in Nursing* 6 (1):1.

Pharmacy Deans Task Force on Professionalism. 2000. White paper on pharmacy student professionalism. *Journal of the American Pharmaceutical Association* 40 (1):96-102.

Pomrehn, P.R., M.V. Davis, D.W. Chen, and W. Barker. 2000. Prevention for the 21st Century: Setting the Context through Undergraduate Medical Education. *Academic Medicine* 75 (7):5S-13.

Robeznieks, A. Feb. 25, 2002. Controlled chaos: Training with surgical simulators. *American Medical News [Online].*

Rosswurm, M.A., and J.H. Larrabee. 1999. A model for change to evidence-based practice. *Image Journal of Nursing Scholarship* 31 (4):317-22.

Scherger, J. March 2002. Informatics. Personal communication to Ann Greiner.

Schillinger, D., M. Wheeler, and A. Fernandez. 2000. The populations and quality improvement seminar for medical residents. *Academic Medicine* 75 (5):562-a, 563.

Self, D.J., M. Olivarez, and D.C. Baldwin, Jr. 1998. The amount of small-group case-study discussion needed to improve moral reasoning skills of medical students. *Academic Medicine* 73 (5):521-23.

Smith, C.A., P.S. Ganschow, B.M. Reilly, A.T. Evans, R.A. McNutt, A. Osei, M. Saquib, S. Surabhi, and S. Yadav. 2000. Teaching residents evidence-based medicine skills: A controlled trial of effectiveness and assessment of durability. *Journal of General Internal Medicine* 15 (10):710-715.

Smith, R.C., J.S. Lyles, J.A. Mettler, A.A. Marshall, L.F. Van Egeren, B.E. Stoffelmayr, G.G. Osborn, and V. Shebroe. 1995. A strategy for improving patient satisfaction by the intensive training of residents in psychosocial medicine: A controlled, randomized study. *Academic Medicine* 70 (8):729-32.

Stead, W. 2002. "Crossing the Quality Chasm: Next Steps for Health Professions Education; Panel Discussion." Online. Available at http://www.kaisernetwork.org/health_cast/hcast_index.cfm?display=detail&hc=601 [accessed Nov. 12, 2002].

Stephenson, K.S., S.M. Peloquin, S.A. Richmond, M.R. Hinman, and C.H. Christiansen. 2002. Changing educational paradigms to prepare allied health professionals for the 21st century. *Education for Health* 15 (1):37-49.

Stumpf, S.H., and J.Z. Clark. 1999. The promise and pragmatism of interdisciplinary education. *Journal of Allied Health* 28 (1):30-32.

Swick, H.M., P. Szenas, D. Danoff, and M.E. Whitcomb. 1999. Teaching professionalism in undergraduate medical education. *Journal of the American Medical Association* 282 (9):830-832.

Taylor, K.J. 2001. Involving nursing students in continuous improvement projects. *Nurse Educator* 26 (4):175-77.

Taylor, R., B. Reeves, P. Ewings, S. Binns, J. Keast, and R. Mears. 2000. A systematic review of the effectiveness of critical appraisal skills training for clinicians. *Medical Education* 34 (2):120-5.

Weeks, W.B., J.L. Robinson, W.B. Brooks, and P.B. Batalden. 2000. Using early clinical experiences to integrate quality-improvement learning into medical education. *Academic Medicine* 75 (1):81-84.

Weissman, D.E., and S.D. Block. 2002. ACGME requirements for end-of-life training in selected residency and fellowship programs: A status report. *Academic Medicine* 77 (4):299-304.

Zwarenstein, M. 1999. A systematic review of interprofessional education. *Journal of Interprofessional Care* 13:417-24.

Chapter 5

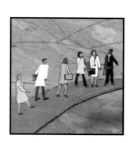

Health Professions Oversight Processes: What They Do and Do Not Do, and What They Could Do

Part of the charge to this committee was to "assess the implications of the changing health system for provider credentialing and licensing programs." The committee interpreted this charge to include the array of mechanisms and rules meant to ensure that health professionals are properly educated and competent to practice. Such mechanisms, grouped by the committee under the rubric of *oversight processes*, include accreditation, licensure, and certification. *Accreditation* serves as a leverage point for the inclusion of particular educational content in academic and continuing education curricula. *Licensure* and *certification* can serve as a lever for ensuring that practicing health professionals meet specific standards and continue to maintain competence in a given content area. The spectrum of oversight processes can also include *organizational accreditation*, which serves to accredit practice institutions and health plans, but has some impact on the continuing competence of practicing professionals through the standards imposed.

This chapter reviews accreditation, licensure, and certification requirements related to the education of health professionals in the five competencies outlined in Chapter 3 with respect to medical, nursing, pharmacy, and physician assistant undergraduates and graduates. A review of all of the allied health professions was beyond the scope of this report. Thus the committee chose to review three allied health occupations that are large and well known, have diverse scopes of authority, collectively include practitioners working in a variety of health care settings, and have an ever-increasing role in caring for the chronically ill: clinical laboratory scientists (also known as medical technologists), occupational therapists, and respiratory therapists. The committee discussed issues related to oversight processes that facilitate or hinder professional development and education in the five competencies and briefly examined the future role of organizational accreditation in fostering the maintenance of competence.

It should be noted that throughout its deliberations, the committee faced a paucity of research in this area. There is virtually no study documenting the impact of accreditation, licensure, or certification on clinician performance or health outcomes.

Overview

The manner in which health professionals are educated and maintain their competence is subject to a myriad of oversight structures and processes, some voluntary and some mandatory. The committee chose to focus on the three primary venues noted above that it believes have the most leverage in determining the initial competency and ongoing professional development and maintenance of competency for practicing clinicians: accreditation, licensure, and certification.

Academic institutions provide learners with opportunities to develop knowledge and skills necessary for safe and effective practice. Ideally, such institutions collaborate with consumers and employers to determine what knowledge and skills are needed for practice. Accrediting organizations assess educational programs to determine whether their content is designed to produce competent graduates and then offer *accreditation* to those programs meeting their standards.

State *licensing* bodies are called upon to protect the public by setting minimum standards of competency for health professionals. They generally do so by establishing educational requirements, assessing character and other attributes, and testing through licensure exams. Health professionals that meet the requirements are granted the right to practice in a given state. Licensing boards interact with health professionals after initial licensure by requiring periodic relicensure or imposing discipline on poor performers. The majority of U.S. health professionals are licensed; thus these boards have a large impact on the ongoing development of health professionals.

Health professional organizations frequently administer or set up independent certifying bodies, which grant a *certification* or credential

recognizing that individuals have successfully demonstrated knowledge of or competency in a particular specialty. Often the requirements for certification go beyond the competency requirements for licensing, which by statute are set to ensure a minimum level of competence. Though the process is usually voluntary, some states mandate certification as part of the licensure process for certain disciplines.

Often professionals work in institutions subject to organizational accreditation. To receive accreditation, such institutions are required to demonstrate that the health professionals they employ or contract with are appropriately skilled. For example, managed care organizations require certification of network clinicians.

It is this patchwork of institutions, all working independently, that defines the nature and length of training for health professionals, their ability to perform particular tasks or work in certain jurisdictions, and the maintenance and development of their skills and competencies.

Educational Accreditation

Educational accreditation, unlike individual licensure and certification, provides evaluation and judgments of institutions and programs rather than individuals. Accreditation guidelines can influence many decisions regarding an educational program, including the number of hours of a particular subject area offered and the types of learning experiences students undertake. If effective, accreditation (Institute of Medicine, 1995):

- Protects the public welfare by ensuring that health professions graduates are appropriately prepared to provide health care services.

- Ensures students that their educational program meets basic standards and facilitates the transfer of credit between different programs.

- Guards public funds from use in support of inferior programs.

- Assists educational programs in achieving—and improving on—minimum standards.

As the roles of the health care workforce have become more specialized over recent decades, a number of new professions have emerged. As a result, many new educational programs have been developed, most having specialized accreditation agencies. Today there are more than 50 health profession accreditation programs (Gelmon et al., 1999). The average educational program is accredited every 3–10 years, with occasional random audits being conducted between accreditation cycles in response to specific problems needing immediate attention.

Standards Related to the Five Competencies

Accrediting organizations vary in their approach to the core competencies, ranging from assessing such competencies in their standards, to requiring related curricula and education experiences, to encouraging educational institutions to include the competencies. Table 5-1 shows how the standards of the various accrediting organizations map to the five competencies set forth in this report.

A number of accrediting bodies have competencies defined in their accreditation standards, representing competencies each deems necessary for practice. These include the accrediting organizations for graduate medicine, pharmacy,[1] and osteopathy; for respiratory therapy; for occupational therapy; and one of the two accrediting bodies for nursing, the National League for Nursing Accrediting Commission (NLNAC). These accrediting bodies require that educational programs offer curricula and educational experiences related to their defined competencies. Within their respective requirements, each addresses selected elements of some or all of the five competencies outlined in this report (see Table 5-1).

Some accreditation organizations do not have articulated competencies that their students should possess upon graduation, but are prescriptive regarding curricula and educational experiences. The accreditation standards for physician assistants, undergraduate medicine, and clinical laboratory have articulated curriculum requirements for those areas deemed integral to the educational preparation of their respective disciplines. These requirements also address certain elements of some of the five competencies (see Table 5-1).

Finally, other accrediting bodies do not have articulated competencies or stated curriculum requirements in their standards. These include the other accrediting body for nursing—the Commission on Collegiate Nursing Education (CCNE)—and that for undergraduate osteopathy. For example, CCNE encourages nursing education programs to pursue teaching, learning, and assessment practices in accordance with the unique mission of the institution — with the aim of supporting flexibility and innovation among institutions — while providing guidance on essential educational elements (American Association of Colleges of Nursing, 1999). However, it does require some evidence of interdisciplinary curricula (Commission on Collegiate Nursing Education, 1998). Such accrediting bodies require that educational programs offer curricula and educational experiences related to their individually defined competencies, which may or may not overlap with the five competencies outlined in this report.

---

[1] The baccalaureate degree is being phased out of pharmacology education. By 2004, all pharmacology programs will offer only the doctor of pharmacy degree.

Table 5-1 Accrediting Organizations and Standards Addressing the Five Competencies

Accrediting Organization	Quality Improvement	Patient-Centered Care	Informatics	Inter-disciplinary Teams	Evidence-Based Practice
Medicine					
Undergraduate					
LCME (Liaison Committee on Medial Education, 2000)		X		X	X
AOA (American Osteopathic Association, 2002b)					
Residency					
ACGME (Accreditation Council for Graduate Medical Education, 1999)	X	X	X	X	X
AOA-Grad (American Osteopathic Association, 2002a)	X	X	X	X	X
Pharmacy					
Undergraduate					
ACPE (American Council on Pharmaceutical Education, 2002)	X	X	X	X	X
Residency					
ASHP (American Society of Health-System Pharmacists, 2001)	X	X	X	X	X
Physician Assistant					
ARC-PA (Accreditation Review Commission on Education for the Physician Assistant, 2001)	X	X	X	X	X
Nursing					
NLNAC (National League for Nursing Accrediting Commission, 1999)		X	X	X	X
CCNE (Commission on Collegiate Nursing Education, 1998)				X	
Occupational Therapy					
ACOTE (Accreditation Council for Occupational Therapy Education, 1998)	X	X	X	X	X
Clinical Laboratory					
NACCLS (National Accrediting Agency for Clinical Laboratory Sciences, 2001)	X		X	X	X
Respiratory Therapy					
C-ARC (Committee on Accreditation for Respiratory Care, 2000)		X	X		X

Accreditation Issues and Debates

Educational Accreditation and Outcomes

At this time, the majority of accrediting organizations are concerned with a descriptive model of evaluating educational programs that focuses on structure and process, such as the number of hours of course content, for a particular subject. A minority of bodies are beginning to expand upon this descriptive model and enlarge their scope to include a focus on evaluating educational institutions based on outcomes (Batalden et al., 2002, Leach, 2002). Outcomes are evidence demonstrating the degree to which the purposes and objectives of an educational program are or are not being attained, including achievement of appropriate skills and competencies by students (Carraccio et al., 2002). Examples of outcomes are learning or development of knowledge, skills, and attitudes by students; improved teaching by faculty; and improved treatment outcomes.

The accrediting bodies surveyed for this report have begun to address outcomes to some extent in their position statements, but vary in their progress toward implementing assessment of educational outcomes. The committee applauds the work of those focusing on outcomes, such as the Accreditation Council for Graduate Medical Education (ACGME) and the American Council on Pharmaceutical Education (ACPE) (see Boxes 5-1 and 5-2) and hopes that other accrediting organizations will follow suit. Many accrediting organizations continue to evaluate programs against process and structure standards, yet there is no research that correlates such an approach with outcomes (Gelmon, 1997).

Box 5-1. Accreditation Council for Graduate Medical Education Competency Requirements

ACGME is shifting from a *descriptive model* for evaluating graduate medical education focused on structure and measured potential to a revised model that measures *accomplishment*. The organization initiated the Outcomes Project in 1997 with the goal of enhancing residency education through residency outcome assessment. While structure will continue to be evaluated as part of the accreditation process, the focus on outcome measures is expected to promote creativity, continuous improvement in both residents and residency programs, and greater public accountability. The Outcomes Project Advisory Group identified the following general competencies for medicine through research and collaborative review:

- *Patient care*—compassionate, appropriate, and effective medical care for the treatment of health problems and the promotion of health.

- *Medical knowledge*—application of established and evolving clinical science to patient care.

- *Practice-based learning and improvement*—incorporation of scientific evidence and improvements into patient care.

- *Interpersonal and communication skills*—teaming with patients, patient families, and other health professionals to provide effective information exchange.

- *Professionalism*—commitment to professional responsibilities, adherence to ethical principles, and sensitivity to diverse patient populations.

(Continued on page 102)

(Continued from page 101)

- *Systems-based practice*—awareness of and responsiveness to the larger context and system of health care and an ability to effectively call on system resources to provide optimal care.

The ACGME Residency Review and Institutional Review Committees have begun integrating general competencies into their requirements, with full integration of defined competencies expected by July 2006.

Sources: Accreditation Council for Graduate Medical Education (2001); Reisdorff et al. (2001).

Box 5-2. American Council on Pharmaceutical Education Competency Requirements

During the last decade, pharmacy education has undergone a major reform to better prepare pharmacy students to provide more patient-centered, outcomes-oriented pharmacy care. Providing such care requires the pharmacist to work in concert with the patient and the patient's other health care providers to promote health; to prevent disease; and to assess, monitor, initiate, and modify medication use. From 1989 through 1993, the American Association of Colleges of Pharmacy (AACP) Commission to Implement Change in Pharmaceutical Education advanced major reforms supporting this vision and specified recommendations regarding the education of pharmacy students, the length of the curriculum, and the appropriate title of the degree granted. As a result, the academic community has shifted from the baccalaureate degree toward adopting the Pharm.D. as the sole professional degree in pharmacy. This reform was further advanced by the AACP Center for the Advancement of Pharmaceutical Education (CAPE) in its development of *Educational Outcomes,* a guide for pharmacy faculty and administrators in assessing and revising their curricula to meet this objective.

The Accreditation Council on Pharmaceutical Education (ACPE) utilized this work in its revision of *Accreditation Standards and Guidelines for the Professional Program in Pharmacy Degree* in 1997. The goals and objectives of the curriculum in pharmacy are now focused on a revised scope of contemporary practice responsibilities, as well as emerging roles that ensure the rational use of drugs in the individualized care of patients and in patient populations. All colleges of pharmacy are now expected to educate and train pharmacists and ensure student mastery of the following 18 professional competencies:

- Evaluate drug orders or prescriptions, accurately and safely compound drugs in appropriate dosage forms, and package and dispense dosage forms.

- Manage systems for storage, preparation, and dispensing of medicines, and supervise technical personnel who may be involved in such processes.

- Manage and administer a pharmacy and pharmacy practice.

- Apply computer skills and technological advances to practice.

(Continued on page 103)

(Continued from page 102)

- Communicate with health care professionals and patients regarding rational drug therapy, wellness, and health promotion.

- Design, implement, monitor, evaluate, and modify or recommend modifications in drug therapy to ensure effective, safe, and economical patient care.

- Identify, assess, and solve medication-related problems, and provide a clinical judgment as to the continuing effectiveness of individualized therapeutic plans and intended therapeutic outcomes.

- Evaluate patients, and order medications and/or laboratory tests in accordance with established standards of practice.

- Evaluate patient problems, and refer patients to other health professionals as appropriate.

- Administer medications.

- Monitor and counsel patients regarding the purposes, uses, and effects of their medications and related therapy.

- Understand relevant diet, nutrition, and nondrug therapies.

- Recommend, counsel in, and monitor patient use of nonprescription drugs.

- Provide emergency first care.

- Retrieve, evaluate, and manage professional information and literature.

- Use clinical data to optimize therapeutic drug regimens.

- Collaborate with other health professionals.

- Evaluate and document interventions and pharmaceutical care outcomes.

Sources: American College of Clinical Pharmacy (2000); Byrd (2002)

The committee recognizes that outcomes-based accreditation is a large challenge and that there are debates about the most effective ways to assess such an approach, how it will be paid for, and how it will be incorporated into accreditation site visits. Regardless, the committee believes that accrediting organizations must surmount these obstacles and begin to move away from the evaluation of programs against process and structure standards, as there is no research that correlates such an approach with improved learning or health outcomes (Gelmon, 1997). The "minimal threshold model," in which the accreditation evaluation serves to identify whether a program has the potential to educate students, is not robust enough to guarantee that students will be competent upon graduation (Accreditation Council for Graduate Medical Education, 2001).

Facilitation of Interdisciplinary Teams

Though accreditation processes vary regarding requirements for the five competencies in the educational experiences of health professionals, accreditation as it is structured today poses a particular barrier to working in interdisciplinary teams at the educational level. A great deal of collaboration and coordination among the various accreditors will be needed to realize the promise of interdisciplinary education. Standards, measures, and incentives for faculty are just some of the matters that need to be aligned by accrediting bodies.

Review bodies have argued that various professions and organizations could benefit greatly from collaboration in developing, testing, and evaluating common core competencies that utilize the same language so that professionals can better communicate and collaborate, with the ultimate goal of improving the quality of care (Health Resources and Services Administration, 1999). Such bodies have argued that many skills are currently taught discipline-by-discipline, whereas these skills often are, or should be, generic to all disciplines. Identifying these skills and collaborating across professions would increase the efficiency with which education is delivered. The Pew Commission for Allied Health expanded this notion by advocating a core curriculum or set of interdisciplinary courses, clinical training, and other educational experiences designed to provide students at each level with common knowledge, skills, and values necessary to perform effectively in the evolving health care workplace (Finocchio et al., 1995; Gelmon, 1997).

Development of a core curriculum or competencies has obvious application to all the health professions. However, it requires extensive collaboration across the existing accrediting organizations and involves working with faculty, professional associations, students, and practicing professionals to determine the content of such curriculum and appropriate standards as benchmarks for educational practice (Gelmon, 1997). Such is not the current reality in the accrediting of health professions schools, though it has been accomplished successfully in health services administration (Gelmon et al., 1990) and public health (Council on Education for Public Health, 1994; Evans and Keck, 1998).

Licensure

The general public does not have adequate information to judge provider qualifications or competence; thus professional licensure laws are enacted to assure the public that practitioners have met the qualifications and minimum competencies required for practice (Safriet, 1994). State governments, through state health professional licensing boards, provide health professionals with the legal authority to practice through licensure. Because licensure is implemented at the state level, there is a great deal of variation in who is licensed and what standards for licensure and practice are applied. State licensure is intended to permit regulations to be tailored to meet local needs, resources, and public expectations, and many boards have public members to ensure that this tailoring is done. Licensing boards evaluate when a health professional's conduct or ability to practice warrants modification, suspension, or revocation of the license. To be licensed, licensees must pass an examination— sometimes national, sometimes administered by the state, or both—that serves to demonstrate that they have acquired basic knowledge for competent practice.

A key licensing issue that affects the health care workforce and the way it is prepared and used is scope-of-practice acts, implemented at the state level. These acts set forth the parameters of practice activities for the licensee, including what duties can be performed, in what settings the licensee can practice, and what (if any) oversight is required. These acts vary tremendously by state, sometimes by location within a state (i.e., rural or urban), and by the types of medical conditions professionals are allowed to treat. All health professions, largely with the exception of medicine, have scopes of practice that limit what they can do to some extent (Jost, 1997; Safriet, 1994). In the case of nurse practitioners, for example, 43 states and the District of Columbia authorize practice through a state board of nursing, and of these, about half have statutory requirements for physician collaboration or supervision and considerable variation in prescriptive authority (Pearson, 2000; Phillips et al., 2002; Safriet, 2002).

Licensure Exams and the Five Competencies

The committee reviewed national licensure examinations for content related to the five competencies. In doing so, the committee kept in mind that schools use the passing rate for such national exams as an educational outcome indicator. Thus the influence of the exam on curricular decisions for educational institutions cannot be underestimated.

All the exams in nursing, pharmacy, and medicine have some content on providing patient-centered care. In allopathic medicine, the licensing exam contains content related to gender, ethnic, and behavioral considerations affecting disease treatment and prevention; psychological and social factors influencing patient behavior; patient interviewing and consultation; and interaction with the family. The osteopathic licensing exam and the physician assistant exam cover health promotion and health prevention content. The computerized licensure exam for registered nurses includes content on psychosocial integrity, communication with the patient, knowledge of and sensitivity to the beliefs and values of the patient, the impact of diversity on the health care experience, and promotion of self-management. The pharmacy licensure exam has content on providing information to patients, including information regarding nutrition, lifestyle, and other nondrug measures that are effective in promoting health.

Some but not all of the licensing exams cover the other competencies. The exams for allopathic medicine and pharmacy cover content related to evidence-based practice, such as interpreting results based on experimental or biometric data, recognizing design features of clinical studies, understanding issues regarding the validity of research protocols, knowing the sensitivity and specificity of selected tests, and recognizing potential bias in clinical studies. The exams for allopathic medicine and registered nurses include content on quality improvement, such as assessment, analysis, planning, implementation and evaluation, error prevention, and safety maintenance. Only the registered nursing exam has content on

interdisciplinary teams. None of the exams has content related to informatics.

In the three allied health disciplines examined, clinical laboratory technologists/ scientists are not uniformly required to be licensed by all states, and thus each state administers its own licensure exams. In occupational therapy, some but not all states require passing the national certification examination administered by the National Board for Certification in Occupational Therapy. That exam has content related to patient-centered skills, especially eliciting patients' values and concerns, making shared decisions, and conducting health promotion, as well as evidence-based practice skills, such as collecting and assessing data from research studies. The exam also covers content related to assessment of service delivery and the collection of satisfaction data related to quality improvement. There is no mention of informatics or interdisciplinary teams. For respiratory therapists, some but not all states require the National Board for Respiratory Care's Entry Level or Advanced Practitioner Respiratory Care examination, which is technical in nature and does not include content related to any of the five competencies.

Table 5-2 shows how the licensing exams in each of the health professions examined by the committee map to the five competencies.

Table 5-2   Licensure Examinations and Content Related to the Five Competencies

Examination	Quality Improvement	Patient-Centered Care	Informatics	Inter-disciplinary Teams	Evidence-Based Practice
Medicine					
USMLE (United States Medical Licensing Exam, 2002a)	X	X			X
COMLEX (National Board of Osteopathic Medical Examiners, 2002)		X			
PANCE (National Commission on Certification of Physician Assistants, 2002)		X			
Pharmacy					
NAPLEX (National Association of Boards of Pharmacy, 2002)		X			X
Nursing					
NCLEX-RN (National Council of State Boards of Nursing, 2000)	X	X		X	
Allied Health					
NCBOT (National Board for Certification in Occupational Therapy, 2002a)	X	X			X
NBRC (National Board for Respiratory Care, 2001)					

Requirements for Maintenance of Licensure

Requirements for maintaining one's clinical license differ from state to state within a given profession, as well among the health professions. In general, one maintains his or her license by paying a fee at the time of license renewal. For certain professions, some states require licensees to take specified hours of continuing education as a condition of relicensure. A recent survey of 323 licensing boards representing a variety of health disciplines revealed that 83 percent required licensees to demonstrate that they had done something to keep their knowledge and skills updated as a condition of license renewal; 94 percent of these boards required licensees to accumulate a specific number of continuing education credits as the only method for doing so (Swankin, 2002).

Regarding the professions reviewed in this paper, the range is great. In pharmacy and occupational therapy, nearly all state boards require that registered professionals complete a certain number of continuing education units before they can renew their licenses (Council on Credentialing in Pharmacy, 2000; Fisher, 2000; National Board for Certification in Occupational Therapy, 2002b). For physician assistants, maintenance of certification from the National Commission on Certification of Physician Assistants is required by 22 state boards as assurance of continued competence (National Commission on Certification of Physician Assistants, 2002), while the other states vary in this regard. In nursing, the majority of boards require only a fee or a certain number of practice hours for maintenance of licensure, with a minority of boards requiring continuing education (Yoder-Wise, 2002).

Licensure Issues and Debates

A review of state licensing laws and related practice acts that define what services health professionals can be licensed to provide was beyond the scope of this report. The committee believes, however, that geographic licensure and scope-of-practice acts may have an effect on the integration of the core competencies—particularly informatics and interdisciplinary teams—into practice and education, and therefore deserve particular attention and further study.

The broad variation among the states in who is licensed and what standards for licensure and practice are applied is one of the trademarks of the licensure system, aimed at ensuring that licensure is tailored to meet local needs, resources, and patient expectations. This approach works well when the health facility, the health professional, and the patient are in the same geographic location. However, the current approach to licensure is increasingly being questioned given the growth of electronic health care and the formation of large, multistate provider groups or teams that cut across geographic boundaries (Finocchio et al., 1998).

When professionals are not practicing in the same state, licensure currently acts as a barrier for many clinical applications of electronic health care that can serve the public's needs. Examples are centralized consultation services to support primary care; the provision of online, continuous, 24-hour monitoring and clinical management of patients in intensive care units for hospitals; and specialty consultations for rural hospitals that do not have such specialists in their communities (Daly, 2000; Hutcherson, 2001; Rosenfeld et al., 2000).

Additionally, the separate scopes of practice, governance structures, and standards maintained by licensing bodies for different types of health professionals—even though these professionals may perform a subset of overlapping functions—as well as the complexity of rules across disciplines and settings, may make it a challenge to form multidisciplinary teams and provide optimum care for patients when they need it (Finocchio et al., 1998; Institute of Medicine, 1996, 2001; Jost, 1997; Sage and Aiken, 1997). Efforts to change scope-of-practice acts are often the focus of turf battles among the professions

fought out in state legislatures; the result is distrust and hostility among professions that are supposed to be collaborating to provide coordinated care (Sage and Aiken, 1997).

Boundaries defined by scope-of-practice acts are sometimes blurred. Studies of diverse physician assistants, nurses, and allied health professionals indicate that they can perform some of the clinical tasks of physicians and provide equivalent quality of care (Kinnersley, 2000; Mundinger et al., 2000; Phillips et al., 2002; Venning, 2000). One panelist at the summit, Charles Inlander of the People's Medical Society, noted: "We still have laws that are so archaic that they protect no one except certain professional bases. That's archaic in this era of technology and better training. It's time for a new look at regulating, and if we do that, we will then be able to focus back on where professional education has to go (Inlander, 2002)."

The committee believes that in today's environment — with care delivery that crosses state lines supported by information technology, more emphasis on interdisciplinary teams, and workforce shortages — licensure and scope-of-practice acts need to be reexamined to ensure that they are flexible enough to allow health professionals to practice to the fullest extent of their technical training and ability. Specifically, health professionals should not be denied the opportunity to realize the promise of optimum patient care offered by utilizing informatics and working in teams.

One example of licensure-supported collaboration for quality care is the increasing number of collaborative practice agreements between physicians and pharmacists (Ferro et al., 1998). Voluntary collaborative practice agreements are characterized by an interdisciplinary approach toward patient care among health care practitioners, allowing pharmacists to extend the provision of pharmaceutical care to the management of various therapies for patients. Depending on the agreement and state regulations or practice acts, pharmacists are able to approve refills, administer drugs and vaccines, and initiate or modify certain types of therapies (American Pharmacuetical Association, 2002). Twenty-seven states now have some form of legislation allowing such an agreement, and in states that have provisions for pharmacists to prescribe, oversight is provided jointly by the medical and pharmacy boards.

To facilitate flexibility and collaboration among certain health professionals, some have proposed multistate or nationally uniform scopes of practice (O'Neil and the Pew Health Professions Commission, 1998) or national licensing systems instead of state-level examinations (Federation of State Medical Boards, 1998). The committee does not recommend one approach over another, but does call for further study to understand these issues, and greater coordination and communication among professional boards both within and across states as the issues are resolved over time. An example of such coordination is described in Box 5-3.

Certification

In contrast with licensure, which is a statutory or regulatory requirement, certification is a voluntary process that is meant to confer recognition of clinical excellence. However, some states mandate certification as part of the licensure process for certain disciplines.[2] Professional organizations grant certification or specialty credentials to practitioners who voluntarily meet additional requirements, such as completing advanced education and training or passing a certifying examination beyond the minimum competencies required for licensure, thus ensuring that they meet the highest standards in an area of specialization (Grossman, 1998). In medicine, where almost 90 percent of physicians are certified by the American Board of Medical Specialties (ABMS), certification is particularly influential in ongoing educational development of physicians. Certification is less influential in pharmacy, where 10 percent of practitioners obtain specialty certification.

Box 5-3. Nurse Licensure Compact

The National Council of State Boards of Nursing has endorsed a mutual recognition model for interstate nursing practice that retains state licensure authority but provides a mechanism for practice across state lines. Such an agreement (or compact) is similar to that among states to honor drivers' licenses. The mutual recognition model of nurse licensure allows a nurse to have one license in his or her state of residency and to practice in other states. When two states have entered into the compact, practice across state lines is allowed unless the nurse is under discipline or a monitoring agreement that would restrict practice. This recognition applies to electronic as well as physical practice.

Advantages of the nurse licensure compact include a reduction in barriers to interstate practice, improvement in tracking for disciplinary purposes, cost-effectiveness and simplicity for the licensee, and facilitation of interstate commerce. Thus far, 15 states have entered into the Nurse Licensure Compact: Arizona, Arkansas, Delaware, Idaho, Iowa, Maine, Maryland, Mississippi, Nebraska, North Carolina, North Dakota, South Dakota, Texas, Utah, and Wisconsin. Other states have compact legislation pending. An up-to-date list of compact states can be found at www.ncsbn.org.

Sources: Finocchio et al. (1998); National Council of State Boards of Nursing (2000).

---

[2] For example, nurse midwives, nurse anesthetists, nurse practitioners, and physician assistants are required to be certified in order to maintain their legal approval to practice in most if not all states.

Content of Certification Examinations Related to the Five Competencies

Initial certification is usually obtained through a one-time examination. The committee reviewed certification requirements and examinations for evidence of content related to the five competencies. It should be noted that the specific content of exam questions can change from year to year and is dependent on the makeup of the committee assigned by the practice organizations to design the test questions (Institute of Medicine, 2002).

As there are a multitude of organizations granting certification in all of the professions, it is difficult to make an assessment of their respective exams. In nursing alone, there are almost 20 organizations that carry out certification, offering nearly 100 specialty certification exams. In general, certification exams are focused primarily on a particular specialty area of practice within a profession.

A review of several certification exams in medicine and pharmacy shows that the majority include content in the area of patient-centered care skills, such as prevention and pain management, as well as evidence-based practice, interdisciplinary teams, and quality improvement. However, they do not include content in informatics (Board of Pharmaceutical Specialties, 2002; Commission for Certification in Geriatric Pharmacy, 2002; National Institute for Standards in Pharmacist Credentialing, 2002).

Requirements for Maintenance of Certification

Certifying bodies are more consistent than licensing boards in their requirements of professionals in that nearly all require some form of evidence of continued competence. While many still rely primarily on continuing education, more and more of these organizations are moving toward other methods of demonstrating continuing competence. In a recent survey of certification bodies from diverse health professions, it was found that 95

percent of the 44 respondents required that their practicing members periodically demonstrate their competency. On average, 86 percent of these organizations offered two or more methods for doing so, including taking approved continuing education courses, retaking the initial certifying exam, and participating in an onsite practice review (Swankin, 2002).

Of the professions reviewed for this report, most but not all mandate periodic recertification, usually by requiring certificate holders to retake the initial certification exam or take a certain number of hours of continuing education, or both (American Board of Medical Specialties, 2000; American Osteopathic Association, 2002b; Commission for Certification in Geriatric Pharmacy, 2002; National Commission on Certification of Physician Assistants, 2002; National Institute for Standards in Pharmacist Credentialing, 2002; Yoder-Wise, 2002). Apart from continuing education and exams, certain pharmacy specialties and occupational therapy offer various paths for recertification, including peer review, self-evaluation, and portfolio review (Board of Pharmaceutical Specialties, 2002; Swankin, 2002). Box 5-4 describes a Canadian model for maintenance of certification.

Organizational Accreditation

This report does not focus directly on organizational accreditors, which accredit practice institutions and health plans. Nonetheless, the committee believes these organizations play an increasing role in ensuring the continued competence of practicing professionals and thus warrant mention. Increasingly, organizational accreditors are, directly or indirectly, specifying educational requirements for individual health professionals. The largest institutional accreditor, the Joint Commission on Accreditation of Healthcare Organizations (JCAHO), which evaluates and accredits more than 17,000 health care organizations and programs in the United States, requires all accredited organizations to assess, prove, track, and improve the competence of all their employees. JCAHO competency standards include the provision of ongoing in-service and other education and training to maintain and improve staff competence, regular collection of data on competence patterns and trends, and identification of and response to staff learning needs (Joint Commission on Accreditation of Healthcare Organizations, 2000). The National Committee for Quality Assurance (NCQA) (2002), which accredits managed care organizations, requires accredited organizations to credential the professionals whom they employ or who practice under their auspices.

Such organizations also have standards related to how care is delivered and performed, with direct implications for clinicians' ongoing professional development. This is particularly the case with regard to quality improvement and patient safety standards. NCQA's accreditation standards specifically mandate quality improvement activities in which practitioners

and health plans are required to participate. Such activities must address data collection, measurement, and analysis to assess performance on three nonpreventive acute or chronic care clinical issues, including one behavioral health issue. Practitioners are also required to participate in the selection and adoption of evidence-based clinical guidelines (National Committee for Quality Assurance, 2002). Patient safety is addressed as well through a standard that requires plans to develop systems to monitor for drug interactions, Food and Drug Administration alerts, and drug recalls, and to alert pharmacists, patients, and providers to potentially serious problems (National Committee on Quality Assurance, 2002). Similarly, JCAHO requires hospitals to initiate specific efforts to prevent medical errors and to tell patients when they have been harmed during their treatment (Joint Commission on Accreditation of Healthcare Organizations, 2001).

Such standards have the potential to serve

Box 5-4. Mandatory Maintenance of Certification Model

The **Royal College of Physicians and Surgeons of Canada** (RCPSC) created a mandatory Maintenance of Certification (MOC) system in 2001 for its fellows—certified specialists in good standing who have applied for admission to fellowship and gained the privilege of using the designation Fellow of the Royal College of Physicians of Canada (FRCPC) or Fellow of the Royal College of Surgeons of Canada (FRCSC). Fellowship, unlike certification, depends on maintaining a process of continued learning.

The RCPSC facilitates the MOC program through a versatile array of learning and reporting portfolios. There are six categories of accreditable activities: accredited group learning; other learning activities (e.g., MEDLINE searches, reading of medical journals); self-assessment programs; practice review and appraisal; and educational development, teaching, and research (e.g., publishing articles, setting standards). The system awards points to fellows for performing such activities, and fellows must obtain at least 400 credit points for every 5-year cycle. Fellows report on their own activities and are encouraged to earn extra credits by putting what they have learned into practice. More points are awarded if outcome studies are conducted on the results of the new practices. Fellows who fail to comply can no longer use the fellowship title. The college plans to publish a public register of fellows who comply in January 2006, and this should have significant implications for employment and practice income. The college will conduct random checks on 3 percent of fellows to audit authenticity.

Source: The Royal College of Physicians and Surgeons of Canada (2002).

---

as a lever for maintenance of competence, though questions remain about their implementation. For example, the JCAHO standards do not dictate how the accredited organization must assess and validate the ongoing competence of its employees. It is up to the individual organizations to determine how their competency programs will be structured. JCAHO surveyors also do not define competence beyond job skills, knowledge, and tasks. Thus, conducting skilled interpersonal communication, acknowledging patient values and promoting shared decision making, being a lifelong learner, applying critical thinking, being an effective team member, and managing information are just some of the many important skills overlooked by such an approach (Decker, 1999; Decker et al., 1997).

Demonstration and Maintenance of Competence

Increasingly, oversight organizations are being challenged to provide assurance to the public that health professionals meet minimum levels of competence throughout their careers, not only at the time of entry and initial licensure and certification. In medicine, surveys have shown that an estimated 20 to 50 percent of primary care practitioners are not aware of or not using new evidence related to common current practices. Yet health professionals face increasing pressures to keep up to date with the ever-expanding knowledge base and new technological innovations, and ongoing knowledge and skill development are necessary to ensure the continued relevance of their clinical care to the changing health care environment.

Currently, there is no mechanism for ensuring that practitioners remain up to date with current best practices. Responsibility for assessing competence is dispersed among multiple authorities. For example, a licensing board may question competence only if it receives a complaint, but most boards do not routinely assess competency after initial licensure. Professional societies and

organizations may require examination for certification and are now beginning to assess competence in addition to knowledge, but such practices are at an early stage and inconsistent among the professions. Some institutional accreditors require competence to be measured for all individual practitioners, but such requirements remain highly task-specific and subject to great variability in terms of implementation in hospitals, health plans, and other health care organizations.

Though the public and professionals themselves might agree that continued competence is desirable, there is much disagreement and debate as to what constitutes evidence of competence, who should ensure it, and how often it should be demonstrated (Grossman, 1998). Historically, licensure has been concerned with minimum competency, whereas certification has been reserved for those meeting higher standards. This distinction is less clear-cut today; for some professions, such as nurse anesthetist, nurse practitioner, and physician assistant, certification adheres to the basic entry standards traditionally required by licensure. Determining where to place the emphasis in reform is further complicated by a lack of research on the effect of certification and licensure on a provider's performance over time (Bashook et al., 2000; Davis et al., 2001).

Evidence of Competence

Though they remain the dominant method used by oversight organizations to assess a health professional's continued competence, traditional, didactic methods of continuing education, such as formal conferences, lectures, and dissemination of educational materials, have been shown to have little effect by themselves on changing clinician behaviors or health outcomes (Cantillon and Jones, 1999; Davis et al., 1999; Davis et al., 1995). Weekend or day courses at hotels or resorts or sessions at professional conferences are viewed more as mini-vacations than as structured learning activities. Indeed, there is widespread and growing consensus that continuing education courses, unless they are based on a needs assessment and require participants to take a test at the end of the course or otherwise demonstrate mastery of the course content, are not a viable means of ensuring that practitioners remain competent over the course of years of practice. To change professional performance and practice, health professionals need to select a portfolio of continuing education activities based on reflection upon the gap between what they know now and what they need to know, not what is just merely convenient or interesting to take. An example of such an approach is presented in Box 5-5.

The Council of Medical Specialty Societies (CMSS) recently convened a task force to review the continuing education field as it presently stands and propose recommendations for reform. Though the task force was addressing the continuing education of medical specialists, its recommendations could be applied to any discipline. The task force recommended that continuing education providers define a core curriculum of content; address competencies; emphasize quality improvement using an evidence-based approach; offer constituents a variety of educational formats; and apply methods to demonstrate the linkage between continuing education and changes in knowledge, skills, clinician practice behaviors, and patient outcomes (Council of Medical Specialty

Societies, 2002).

Research also suggests that lecture-based courses need to be reinforced with interactive techniques, such as case discussion, role play, and hands-on practice sessions, offering a chance to apply the new knowledge or skills in practice, and then reinforce these activities with further educational sessions (Davis et al., 1999; O'Brien et al., 2001). Research suggests further that continuing education needs to emphasize a variety of interventions, particularly reminder systems, academic detailing, and patient-mediated methods, and to use a mix of approaches, including Web-based technologies (Cantillon and Jones, 1999; O'Brien et al., 2001; Smith, 2000). William Stead, Vanderbilt University, suggested at the summit in his address:

> We have begun to experiment with some forms of continuing education that may be more effective....You can watch [health providers'] pattern of intervention with the system, and you can identify areas in which they have need for information, and then deliver this in a tailored educational intervention. Another thing you can really begin to do is take those same tools and use them in a case-based learning experience, where you present people with a

---

Box 5-5. Continuing Education System in Dietetics

The Commission on Dietetic Registration (CDR) recently required that a Professional Development Portfolio be part of its recertification process for certificate holders. By 2006, all registered dieticians and dietetic technicians will be recertifed using this new process. Under the portfolio approach, the dietician submits a portfolio for CDR approval, outlining his or her plan for reflection and assessment of learning needs, development of a learning plan, self-evaluation of learning plan objectives, and application of learning activities that have a direct relationship to his or her needs. Learning activities include structured courses, professional leadership, sponsored independent learning (e.g., mentoring relationships), and reading from professional journals. CDR provides tools for self-directed learning and verifies that steps in the process have been completed and meet minimum guidelines. CDR is auditing such portfolios at random by identified triggers.

Source: Commission on Dietetic Registration (2002).

simulated problem and let them use the information tools to work through it. I think the biggest thing we've got to do with continuing education is to make it model problem solving, instead of being a separate event that's taken out of the work process. (Stead, 2002)

The committee perceives a larger issue with continuing education—the lack of relevance of the content of existing courses to providing care that meets the health care needs of the population. There is no formalized process that ensures coverage of the five competencies outlined in Chapter 3. Some licensing boards require that health professionals choose specific courses for maintenance of their license, but more often than not, the choice is wide open, and health care practitioners can select a course that is merely interesting or even just convenient.

Measurement of Competence

Computerized or written multiple-choice examinations are the main method by which professionals are initially licensed or certified. Questions remain about the validity of this approach (Epstein and Hundert, 2002). Some licensure and certification exams do not encompass the range of complexity and degree of uncertainty encountered in practice, or the psychosocial behaviors needed for practice. In medicine, both the licensing and certification exams are being revised to include more psychometric measures. By mid-2004, the United States Medical Licensing Exam is scheduled to include a new provision requiring graduates to demonstrate that they can gather information from patients, perform a physical examination, and communicate their findings to patients and colleagues. This exam is currently required only for international medical graduates. To "pass" the examination, a candidate must demonstrate both satisfactory clinical skills and satisfactory communication skills, including providing feedback and counseling to the patient (United States Medical Licensing Exam, 2002b).

A variety of other mechanisms—peer review, professional portfolio, objective structured clinical examination, patient survey, record review, and patient simulation—also are being explored by certification bodies, and to some extent by licensing boards, as means of assessment. These have been shown to be valid measures of professional performance, and the consensus is that a combination of such approaches is the best strategy (Epstein and Hundert, 2002; Murray et al., 2000). Box 5-6 presents one example of such an integrated approach to professional development.

Conclusion

Ultimately, accreditation, certification, and licensure are collectively but one leverage point for ensuring that health professionals maintain up-to-date skills and competencies. Educational institutions have an essential part to play in instilling a sense of the importance of being a lifelong learner, and employers also have a major role in shaping the ongoing professional development of health professionals. However, the oversight system remains a critical lever, and there is room for improvement in the system with regard to ongoing competency development.

Lifelong learning can be thought of in six stages, each impacted by the oversight system. Upon entering academic education, health professionals are considered to be at the novice stage. As they progress through educational programs and complete their professional education, which is based on explicit, measurable outcome measures set forth in accreditation standards, they are considered to be at the advanced beginner stage. After completing their academic experiences and residency and internship as relevant, they obtain licensure and/or certification based on defined measures and are at the competent stage of the learning process. As they progress through their careers, they enter the proficient stage through repeated experiences and ongoing maintenance of competence by means of assessment and feedback provided by peers, licensing boards, employers, and certification bodies. In the expert stage, midcareer professionals have learned to recognize patterns of discrete clues and to work quickly with better intuition (Batalden et al., 2002). Ultimately, health professionals who remain lifelong learners, continuously updating their skills and knowledge, accumulating more and more practice hours in their field, and supported by an oversight system that provides regular feedback on their performance, arrive at the master stage of the learning process.

In the majority of the professions, however, there is no formal oversight group to ensure a smooth, organized progression of education through these stages. Educational programs and accreditation, certification, and licensure bodies all work separately and sometimes at odds, and are at times reviewing the same elements (Enarson and Burg, 1992; Ludmerer, 1999). For example, in nursing, schools are approved twice: the majority of states require that a postsecondary educational program have state licensing board approval if it is to apply for accreditation by one of the two nursing accreditation bodies—NLNAC or CCNE. In medicine, for example, the following organizations all influence the content of medical education: the Liaison Committee on Medical Education, the Association of

American Medical Colleges, the Accreditation Council for Graduate Medical Education, 27 residency review committees, ABMS and its 24 certifying boards, the Bureau of Health Professions at the Department of Health and Human Services, the American Medical Association, the American Osteopathic Association and its 18 certifying boards, the American Association of Colleges of Osteopathic Medicine, and various professional societies involved in continuing medical education (Institute of Medicine, 2001).

Because so many health professionals must graduate from an accredited program in order to sit for licensure exams and obtain specialty certification, greater linkage among accreditation, certification, and licensure is imperative. It means very little if accreditation standards impose on educational programs requirements that are not reinforced in the licensing exam. All processes must be linked so they are focused on the same outcome—the competence of the professional to deliver quality health care. Accomplishing this linkage requires partnerships among licensing and accreditation boards, certification programs, and educational institutions. Summit panelist Joey Ridenour, National Council of State Boards of Nursing, concurred: "I think one of the strategies that would be most important for us as

---

Box 5-6. American Board of Internal Medicine and Continuous Professional Development

In 2000, the American Board of Internal Medicine (ABIM) introduced a recertification process that builds on the current knowledge-centered program by adding assessments of clinical and communication skills, clinical performance, and medical outcomes, based on the four competencies recommended by ABMS for maintenance of certification. The three-part process, termed a program of continuous professional development, includes self-evaluation exercises, documentation of essential knowledge, and confirmation of satisfactory qualifications and professional and community good standing. The process includes examination of knowledge, verification of credentials, and completion of at least five self-assessment exercises: two assessing practice outcomes, one assessing new knowledge, one assessing clinical skills (physical diagnosis and communication), and one assessing professionalism (doctor–patient relationship and patient care).

Sources: ABIM Foundation (2002); Wasserman et al. (2000).

---

regulators is to continue to work together among disciplines to identify…competencies that people need to develop over time, and continue to discuss how these will be played out…not only in traditional but in continuing education (Ridenour, 2002)." Also, as noted earlier, since professionals are increasingly called upon to provide care that crosses state lines and care in interdisciplinary teams, geographic licensure and scope-of-practice acts must be examined to determine whether modification is necessary to promote this type of care.

Though many agree that some form of continued competence is important, health professionals and experts struggle with how to test competency and who should be involved in competency assurance. A lack of resources and political tensions among the various organizations are major barriers to the assurance of continued competence. Moreover, the complexity of the health care environment and the vast differences in practice make testing for competence difficult, as areas of expertise may not fit well with standardized testing (Whittaker et al., 2000).

In summary, the committee's assessment of the oversight environment leads to the following conclusions.

Accreditation

- **There is little evidence to suggest that accreditation status has a significant influence on health professionals' education as regards delivering care that meets patients' needs.**

- **Only a few accrediting bodies require educational programs to assess the competency of their graduates.**

Licensure

- **Geographic licensure restrictions and scope-of-practice acts may impede the ability of practicing professionals to use some electronic applications for health care and to work in interdisciplinary teams. These issues need further examination.**

- **Some licensing boards require periodic demonstration of continued competency, with continuing education being the dominant method for such demonstration.**

- **The singular focus of continuing education as a method to ensure ongoing competence is problematic considering the number of studies indicating that this approach is not effective.**

Certification

- **The majority of certification agencies require periodic demonstration of competency, using continuing education and other methods for such demonstration.**

- **Many certification agencies still rely on continuing education to demonstrate continued competence, but are increasingly moving toward other, more effective methods.**

Organizational Accreditation

- **Organizational accreditors have a role in ensuring the ongoing competency of practicing professions. Standards that exist focus mainly on quality improvement and patient safety.**

References

ABIM Foundation. 2002. Medical professionalism in the new millennium: A physician charter. *Annals of Internal Medicine* 136 (3):243-46.

Accreditation Council for Graduate Medical Education. 1999. "General Competencies." Online. Available at http://www.acgme.org/outcome/comp/compFull.asp [accessed June, 2002].

Accreditation Council for Graduate Medical Education. 2001. "Annual Report 2001." Online. Available at http://www.acgme.org/About/2001AnnRep.pdf [accessed May 31, 2002].

Accreditation Council for Occupational Therapy Education. 1998. "Standards for an Accredited Educational Program for the Occupational Therapist." Online. Available at http://www.aota.org/nonmembers/area13/links/LINK31.asp [accessed Aug. 15, 2002].

Accreditation Review Commission on Education for the Physician Assistant, I.A.-P. 2001 . "Accreditation Standards for the Physician Assistant." Online. Available at http://www.arc-pa.org/General/standards/standards01.pdf [accessed Aug., 2002].

American Association of Colleges of Nursing. 1999. *Essential Clinical Resources for Nursing's Academic Mission.* Washington, DC: AACN.

American Board of Medical Specialties. 2000. "Recertification and Time-Limited Certification." Online. Available at http://www.abms.org/Downloads/General_Requirements/Table6.PDF [accessed Nov., 2002].

American College of Clinical Pharmacy. 2000. A vision of pharmacys future roles, responsibilities, and manpower needs in the United States. *Pharmacotherapy* 20 (8):991-1020.

American Council on Pharmaceutical Education. 2002. "Criteria for Quality and Interpretive Guidelines for Approval of Continuing Pharmaceutical Education ." Online. Available at http://www.acpe-accredit.org/frameset_AppProv.htm [accessed Sept., 2002].

American Osteopathic Association. 2002a. "Postdoctoral Internship and Residency Standards and Procedures." Online. Available at http://www.aoa-net.org/Accreditation/postdoctoral/postdocpdf.htm [accessed 2002a].

American Osteopathic Association. 2002b. "Maintenance of Certification." Online. Available at http://www.aoa-net.org/Certification/maintain.htm [accessed Aug., 2002b].

American Pharmacuetical Association. 2002. "Principles of Practice for Pharmaceutical Care." Online. Available at http://www.aphanet.org/pharmcare/prinprac.html [accessed 2002].

American Society of Health-System Pharmacists. 2001. "The Residency Learning System (RLS) Model ." Online. Available at http://www.ashp.org/public/rtp/Model/model.html [accessed Sept., 2002].

Bashook, P.G., S.H. Miller, J. Parboosingh, and S.D. Horowitz. 2000. "Credentialing Physician Specialists: A World Perspective." Online. Available at http://www.abms.org/Downloads/Conferences/Credentialing%20Physician%20Specialists.pdf [accessed Sept. 15, 2002].

Batalden, P., D. Leach, S. Swing, H. Dreyfus, and S. Dreyfus. 2002. General competencies and accreditation in graduate medical education. *Health Affairs* 21 (5):103-11.

Board of Pharmaceutical Specialties. 2002. "Recertification." Online. Available at http://www.bpsweb.org/BPS/recert-gen.html#top [accessed Sept., 2002].

Byrd, G. 2002. Can the profession of pharmacy serve as a model for health informationist professionals? *Journal of Medical Library Association* 90 (1):68-75.

Cantillon, P., and R. Jones. 1999. Does continuing medical education in general practice make a difference? *British Medical Journal* 318 (7193):1276-79.

Carraccio, C., S.D. Wolfsthal, R. Englander, K. Ferentz, and C. Martin. 2002. Shifting paradigms: From flexner to competencies. *Academic Medicine* 77 (5):361-67.

Commission for Certification in Geriatric Pharmacy. 2002. "Fees and Eligibility Requirements." Online. Available at http://www.ccgp.org/pharmacists/body_fees.htm [accessed Sept., 2002].

Commission on Collegiate Nursing Education. 1998. "Standards for Accreditation of Baccalaureate and Graduate Nursing Education Programs." Online. Available at http://www.aacn.nche.edu/Accreditation/standrds.htm [accessed Aug., 2002].

Commission on Dietetic Registration. 2002. "Professional Development Portfolio Guide." Online. Available at http://www.cdrnet.org/pdrcenter/portfoliotoc.htm [accessed Oct., 2002].

Committee on Accreditation for Respiratory Care. 2000. "Standards and Guidelines for the Profession of Respiratory Care ." Online. Available at http://www.coarc.com/accred/standards.html [accessed Aug. 15, 2002].

Council of Medical Specialty Societies. 2002. "Repositioning the Future of Medical Education." Online. Available at http://www.cmss.org/index.cfm?p=readmore&itemID=1034&detail=Task%20Force%20%2D%20Expert%20Groups [accessed Sept., 2002].

Council on Credentialing in Pharmacy. 2000. "Credentialing in Pharmacy." Online. Available at http://www.pharmacycredentialing.org/ccp/whitepaper.htm [accessed Sept., 2002].

Council on Education for Public Health. 1994. *Accreditation Criteria and Procedures.* Washington, DC: CEPH.

Daly, H.L. 2000. Telemedicine: The invisible legal barriers to the health care of the future. *Annals of Health Law* 9:73-106, inside cover.

Davis, B.E., D.B. Nelson, O.J. Sahler, F.A. McCurdy, R. Goldberg, and L.W. Greenberg. 2001. Do clerkship experiences affect medical students attitudes toward chronically ill patients? *Academic Medicine* 76 (8):815-20.

Davis, D., M.A. OBrien, N. Freemantle, F.M. Wolf, P. Mazmanian, and A. Taylor-Vaisey. 1999. Impact of formal continuing medical education: Do conferences, workshops, rounds, and other traditional continuing education activities change physician behavior or health care outcomes? *Journal of American Medical Association* 282 (9):867-74.

Davis, D.A., M.A. Thomson, A.D. Oxman, and R.B. Haynes. 1995. Changing physician performance. A systematic review of the effect of continuing medical education strategies. *JAMA* 274 (9):700-705.

Decker, P.J. 1999. The hidden competencies of healthcare: Why self-esteem, accountability, and professionalism may affect hospital customer satisfaction scores. *Hospital Topic* 77 (1):14-26.

Decker, P.J., M.K. Strader, and R.J. Wise. 1997. Beyond JCAHO: using competency models to improve healthcare organizations. Part I. *Hospital Topic* 75 (1):23-8.

Enarson, C., and F.D. Burg. 1992. An overview of reform initiatives in medical education. 1906 through 1992. [Review] [22 refs]. *Journal of American Medical Association* 268 (9):1141-43.

Epstein, R.M., and E.M. Hundert. 2002. Defining and assessing professional competence. *Journal of the American Medical Association* 287 (2):226-35.

Evans, P.P., and C.W. Keck. 1998. Accreditation well-established in higher education; offers useful lessons for other arenas. [Review] [9 refs]. *Journal of Public Health Management & Practice.* 4 (4):19-24.

Federation of State Medical Boards. 1998. "Maintaining State-Based Medical Licensure and Discipline: A Blueprint for Uniform and Effective Regulation of the Medical Profession." Online. Available at http://www.fsmb.org/uniform.htm [accessed Jan. 12, 2001].

Ferro, L.A., R.E. Marcrom, L. Garrelts, M.S. Bennett, E.E. Boyd, L. Eddinger, R.D. Shafer, and M.L. Fields. 1998. Collaborative practice agreements between pharmacists and physicians. *J Am Pharm Assoc (Wash)* 38 (6):655-64; quiz 664-6.

Finocchio, L. J., C. M. Dower, N. T. Blick, C. M. Gragnola, and the Taskforce on Health Care Workforce Regulation. 1998. *Strengthening Consumer Protection: Priorities for Health Care Workforce Regulation.* San Francisco, CA: Pew Health Professions Commission.

Finocchio, L.J., C.M. Dower, T. McMahon, C.M. Gragnola, and Task Force on health Care Workforce Regulation. 1995 . *Reforming Health Care Workforce Regulation: Policy Considerations for the 21st Century.* San Francisco, CA: Pew Health Professions Commission.

Fisher, G.S. 2000. Mandatory continuing education: The future of occupational therapy professional development? *Occupational Therapy in Health Care* 13 (2):1-24.

Gelmon, S., E. O'Neil, J. Kimmey, and The Task Force on Accreditation of Health Professions Education. 1999. *Strategies for Change and Improvement: The Report of the Task Force on Accreditation of Health Professions Education.* San Francisco: Center for the Health Professions, University of California at San

Francisco.

Gelmon, S.B. 1997. Accreditation, core curriculum and allied health education: Barriers and opportunities. *Journal of Allied Health* 26 (3):119-25.

Gelmon, S.B., D.M. OBrien, D.A. Conrad, and S.M. Shortell. 1990. Educating healthcare leaders for the 21st century: evolution not revolution. *Healthcare Executives* 5 (1):34-7.

Grossman, J. 1998. Continuing competence in the health professions. *American Journal of Occupational Therapy* 52 (9):709-15.

Health Resources and Services Administration. 1999. *Building the Future of Allied Health: Report of the Implementation Task Force of the National Commission on Allied Health.* Rockville, MD: Health Resources and Services Administration.

Hutcherson, C.M. 2001. "Legal considerations for nurses practicing in a telehealth setting. Online Journal of Issues in Nursing." Online. Available at http://www.nursingworld.org/ojin/topic16/tpc16_3.htm

Inlander, C. 2002. ""Crossing the Quality Chasm: Next Steps for Health Professions Education"; Panel Discussion." Online. Available at http://www.kaisernetwork.org/health_cast/hcast_index.cfm?display=detail&hc=601 [accessed Nov. 12, 2002].

Institute of Medicine. 1995. *Dental Education at a Crossroads.* Vol. Committee on the Future of Dental Education and Marilyn J. Field, eds. Washington, DC: National Academy Press.

———. 1996. *Telemedicine: A Guide to Assessing Telecommunications for Health Care* . Marilyn J. Field, ed. Washington, DC: National Academy Press.

———. 2001. *Crossing the Quality Chasm: A New Health System for the 21st Century.* Washington, DC: National Academy Press.

———. 2002. *Confronting Chronic Neglect: The Education and Training of Health Professionals on Family Violence.* Vol. Committee on the Training Needs of Health Professionals to Respond to Family Violence, Board of Children Youth and Families, Institute of Medicine, and F. Cogn M.E.S.a.J.D.S., Eds. Washington, DC: National Academy Press.

Joint Commission on Accreditation of Healthcare Organizations. 2000. Age-Specific Competencies.

Joint Commission on Accreditation of Healthcare Organizations. 2001. "Hospitals Face New JACHO Patient Safety Standards on July 1." Online. Available at http://www.jcaho.org/news+room/press+kits/hospitals+face+new+jcaho+patient+safety+standards+on+july+1.htm [accessed 2002].

Jost, T. 1997. *Regulation of the Healthcare Professions.* 1997: Health Administration Press.

Kinnersley, P. 2000. Randomised controlled trial of nurse practioner versus general practitioner care for patients requesting same day consultations in primary care. *British Medical Journal* 320 (7241):1043-48.

Leach, D.C. 2002. Building and assessing competence: the potential for evidence-based graduate medical education. Qual Manag Health Care 11(1):39-44.

Liaison Committee on Medial Education. 2000. "Overview of the Accrediation of the LCME." Online [accessed Aug., 2002].

Ludmerer, K. 1999. *Time to Heal: American Medical Education from the Turn of the Century to the Era of Managed Care.* New York, NY: Oxford University Press.

Mundinger, M.O., R.L. Kane, E.R. Lenz, A.M. Totten, W.Y. Tsai, P.D. Cleary, W.T. Friedewald, A.L. Siu, and M.L. Shelanski. 2000. Primary care outcomes in patients treated by nurse practitioners or physicians: A randomized trial. *Journal of the American Medical Association* 283 (1):59-68.

Murray, E., L. Gruppen, P. Catton, R. Hays, and J.O. Woolliscroft. 2000. The accountability of clinical education: Its definition and assessment. *Medical Education* 34 (10):871-79.

National Accrediting Agency for Clinical Laboratory Sciences. 2001. *Standards of Accredited Educational Programs for the Clinical Laboratory Scientist/Medical Technologist.* Chicago, IL: National Accrediting Agency for Clinical Laboratory Sciences.

National Association of Boards of Pharmacy. 2002. "Examinations -- NAPLEX." Online. Available at http://www.nabp.net/ [accessed Aug. 10, 2002].

National Board for Certification in Occupational Therapy. 2002a. "Practice Exams." Online. Available at http://www.nbcot.org/nbcot/docs/practice_exam_web_page.doc [accessed Aug., 2002a].

———. 2002b. "State Regulations." Online. Available at http://www.nbcot.org/nbcot/scripts/state_reg/regulations.asp [accessed Aug., 2002b].

National Board for Respiratory Care. 2001. "Examinations." Online. Available at http://www.nbrc.org/ExamsRRT.htm [accessed Sept., 2002].

National Board of Osteopathic Medical Examiners. 2002. "Guidelines and Sample Exams." Online. Available at http://www.nbome.org/ [accessed 2002].

National Commission on Certification of Physician Assistants. 2002. "Recertification: Overview." Online. Available at http://www.nccpa.net/REC_overview.asp [accessed Aug., 2002].

National Committee for Quality Assurance. 2002. "What Does NCQA Review When It Accredits an HMO?" Online. Available at http://www.ncqa.org/Programs/Accreditation/MCO/mcostdsoverview.htm [accessed 2002].

National Committee on Quality Assurance. 2002. "NCQA Releases Draft 2003 MCO, MBHO, and PPO Standards; Changes Streamline Process, Emphasize Results." Online. Available at http://www.ncqa.org/Communications/News/mcopubcomment2003.htm [accessed 2002].

National Council of State Boards of Nursing. 2000. "Nurse Licensure Compact." Online. Available at http://www.ncsbn.org/public/nurselicensurecompact/mutual_recognition.htm [accessed Aug., 2002].

National Institute for Standards in Pharmacist Credentialing. 2002. "Recertification Requirements and Guidelines." Online. Available at http://www.nispcnet.org/recert_guidelines.pdf [accessed Aug., 2002].

National League for Nursing Accrediting Commission. 1999. "1999 Standards and Criteria and Interpretative Guidelines." Online. Available at http://www.nlnac.org/Manual%20&%20IG/01_accreditation_manual.htm [accessed Aug. 14, 2002].

OBrien, T., N. Freemantle, A.D. Oxman, F. Wolf, D. A. Davis, and J. Herrin. 2001. Continuing education meetings and workshops: Effects on professional practice and health care outcomes. *Cochrane Database System Review* (2): CD003030.

ONeil, E. H. and the Pew Health Professions Commission. 1998. *Recreating health professional practice for a new century - The fourth report of the pew health professions Commission.* San Francisco, CA: Pew Health Professions Commission.

Pearson, L. 2000. Annual legislative update: How each state stands on legislative issues affecting advanced nursing practice. *The Nurse Practitioner* 26 (1):7-57.

Phillips, R.L. Jr, D.C. Harper, M. Wakefield, L.A. Green, and G.E. Fryer, Jr. 2002. Can nurse practitioners and physicians beat parochialism into plowshares? *Health Affairs* 21 (5):133-42.

Reisdorff, E.J., O.W. Hayes, D.J. Carlson, and G.L. Walker. 2001. Assessing the new general competencies for resident education: A model from an emergency medicine program. *Academic Medicine* 76 (7):753-57.

Ridenour, J. 2002. ""Crossing the Quality Chasm: Next Steps for Health Professions Education"; Panel Discussion." Online. Available at http://www.kaisernetwork.org/health_cast/hcast_index.cfm?display=detail&hc=601 [accessed Nov. 12, 2002].

Rosenfeld, B.A., T. Dorman, M.J. Breslow, et al. 2000. Intensive care unit telemedicine: Alternate paradigm for providing continuous intensivist care. *Critical Care Medicine* 28 (12):3925-31.

Safriet, B. 2002. Closing the gap between can and may in health-care providers scopes of practices. *Yale Journal on Regulation* 19 (2):301-34.

Safriet, B.J. 1994. Impediments to progress in health care workforce policy: License and practice laws. *Inquiry* 31 (3):310-317.

Sage, W. M., and L. H. Aiken. 1997. Regulating interdisiplinary practice. *Regulation of the Healthcare Professions.* T. Jost. Chicago: Health Administration Press.

Smith, W.R. 2000. Evidence for the effectiveness of techniques to change physician behavior. *Chest* 118 (2 Suppl):8S-17S.

Stead, W. 2002. "Crossing the Quality Chasm: Next Steps for Health Professions Education; Panel Discussion." Online. Available at http://www.kaisernetwork.org/health_cast/hcast_index.cfm?display=detail&hc=601 [accessed Nov. 12, 2002].

Swankin, D.S. 2002. *Results of Survey of Selected State Health Licensing Boards and Health Voluntary Certification Agencies Concerning their Continuing Competence Programs and Requirements*. Washington, DC: Citizen Advocacy Center.

The Royal College of Physicians and Surgeons of Canada. 2002. "Maintenance of Certification." Online [accessed Oct., 2002].

United States Medical Licensing Exam. 2002a. "United States Medical Licensing Examination - Steps 1, 2, 3." Online. Available at http://www.usmle.org/step1/intro.htm [accessed Aug. 10, 2002a].

———. 2002b. "Frequently Asked Questions About the USMLE Clinical Skills Exam." Online. Available at http://www.usmle.org/news/faqscse.htm [accessed Aug. 10, 2002b].

Venning, P., *et al.* 2000. Randomised controlled trial comparing cost effectiveness of general practitioners and nurse practitioners in primary care. *British Medical Journal* 320 (7241):1048-53.

Wasserman, S.I., H.R. Kimball, and F.D. Duffy. 2000. Recertification in internal medicine: A program of continuous professional development. Task Force on Recertification. *Annals of Internal Medicine* 133 (3):202-8.

Whittaker, S., W. Carson, and M.C. Smolenski. 2000. Assuring continued competence -- policy questions and approaches: How should the profession respond? *Online Journal of Issues in Nursing*:18.

Yoder-Wise, P.S. 2002. State and association/certifying boards: CE requirements. *Journal of Continuing Education in Nursing* 33 (1):3-11.

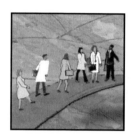

Chapter 6

Recommendations for Reform

This chapter sets forth the committee's recommendations for achieving the following overarching vision for the reform of health professions education to enhance the quality and safety of patient care. This vision—for all programs and institutions engaged in the clinical education of health professionals—encompasses the five competencies that health professionals need in order to practice in the redesigned system described in the *Quality Chasm* report (Institute of Medicine, 2001).

> *All health professionals should be educated to deliver patient-centered care as members of an interdisciplinary team, emphasizing evidence-based practice, quality improvement approaches, and informatics.*

A number of the following 10 recommendations focus on oversight organizations. This is because the committee believes that integrating a core set of competencies—one that is shared across the professions—into health professions oversight processes would provide a good deal of leverage in terms of reform, and is an important first step in aligning incentives and providing a catalyst for both educational institutions and professional associations to make necessary changes. This effort would build upon existing efforts and create synergies across the disciplines. A recent article synthesizing nine major reports on physician competencies appears to support this approach, concluding that "without data about medical-education quality, accreditation is the most potent lever for curricula reform in our decentralized medical education system." (Halpern, 2001)

The committee also recommends pursing other leverage points to reform health professions education—such as the use of report cards that incorporate education-related measures and innovations in financial incentives. However, the preponderance of its recommendations are directed at oversight organizations. This is the case in part because of the lack of education measures and the charge to this committee, which was focused on clinical education.[1] Also, health professions oversight processes, such as accreditation and certification, function at the national level, thereby affording a mechanism for systemwide change. Oversight bodies are diverse, including representation on their boards from professional associations, educational institutions, and consumer representatives, and include both public and private organizations.

The committee believes that a competency-based approach to education could result in better quality because educators would begin to have information on outcomes, which could ultimately lead to better patient care. Defining a core set of competencies across educational oversight processes holds the potential for reducing costs as a result of better communication and coordination across oversight bodies, with processes being streamlined and redundancies reduced. Integrating core competencies into oversight processes would likely provide the impetus for faculty development, curricular reform, and leadership activities. Specifically, academic institutions would add or modify coursework, boards would revise licensing exams, and certifying organizations would seek to respond to the new criteria in their requirements for maintaining competency. The importance of this area was apparent at the Institute of Medicine (IOM) summit, where the oversight working group attracted the largest number of participants and generated the largest number of proposed actions, even though members of oversight bodies represented only about 20 percent of the summit participants (see Appendix B). Moreover, participants identified oversight processes as a primary driver in an exercise aimed at identifying key strategies.

Common Language and Adoption of Core Competencies

Any collective movement by the health professions to reform education must begin with defining a shared language that will enable the professions to communicate and collaborate with one another (Bashook and Parboosingh, 1998; Carraccio et al., 2002; Halpern et al., 2001; Harden, 2002). A synthesis of nine major reports related to curriculum reform and competencies underscores the need for such a shared vocabulary (Halpern et al., 2001), noting that common terms can facilitate the development of new curricula, with departments and programs having a greater ability to coordinate related courses and training activities. A lack of consensus around language and terms related to the five competencies may be hampering their implementation. It may also be undermining attempts to define a core set of competencies across the professions and to integrate these competencies into oversight processes (Lavin et al., 2001; Pomeroy and Philp, 1994).

In the case of evidence-based practice, for example, there is no standardized definition of evidence. The existing definitions include evidence that can be quantified, such as randomized controlled trials; evidence based on qualitative research; evidence that exists in institutional databases; and evidence derived from the knowledge and experience of experts and peers, including inductive reasoning (Guyatt et al., 2000; Higgs et al., 2001; Welch and Lurie, 2000). In recent years, leaders in the field have worked to expand the definition of evidence to include qualitative research and to dispel the myth that evidence-based practice ignores clinical experience and expertise (Guyatt et al., 2000). However, a review of the literature suggests that misunderstanding and misconceptions regarding the definition of evidence persist (Marwick, 2000; Mazurek, 2002; Mitchell, 1999; Satya-Murti, 2000; Woolf, 2000). Some also argue that clinicians must think in terms of hierarchies of evidence and always seek the highest level of available quantifiable evidence to inform their practices (Sackett, 1998). This view concerns some leaders, who argue that such an approach could introduce bias in methodologies and conclusions (Ching, 2002) and further

---

[1] A current Institute of Medicine study addressing academic health centers is considering financing questions.

reinforces a biomedical model that could prevent greater adoption of more holistic views of human health (Shaver, 2002).

A related issue is the implementation of evidence-based practice skills across the professions—particularly as part of a computerized decision support system that supports all clinicians. The problem is that terms and therefore standards for indexing are lacking, making linkages between profession-specific databases difficult. Therefore, each profession's evidence base exists in its own silo (Closs and Cheater, 1999), without the linkages required in an interdisciplinary academic or practice environment (Evers, 2001; Lang, 1999; Prentice and Bentley, 1999). Finally, the lack of common terms may make assessing the evidence base on any given topic difficult (Jordan, 2000).

The lack of consistent language impedes the development of interdisciplinary team skills. Even the term *interdisciplinary* may confuse and confound; in medicine, it can mean working across the medical specialties. A review of the literature related to teaching interdisciplinary team skills reveals differing terminologies as an obstacle: faculty struggle to understand other professions' core concepts and content, and the result may be conflict when developing and teaching interdisciplinary courses (Lavin et al., 2001; Pomeroy and Philp, 1994).

Some argue that to have effective interdisciplinary settings, clinicians must develop a unifying framework for interpreting all types of decisions. For example, Buckingham and Adams (2000) stress the need for the professions to go beyond a framework that describes nurses' clinical decisions as evaluative and physicians' as diagnostic, viewing such distinctions as a barrier to interdisciplinary teams, overlapping roles, and fluidity in role boundaries.

In the area of informatics, there is disagreement about whether the subject needs to be viewed and taught in discipline-specific ways or approached more generically. Some argue that each discipline should require its own core informatics curricula and training programs to best serve the needs of that particular health professions group. Others disagree, asserting that informatics is built upon a reusable and widely applicable set of methods that is common to all health professionals (Masys et al., 2000; Raymond H. Curry et al., 2000).

Dan Duffy, American Board of Internal Medicine, acknowledged the lack of consistent language at the summit:

> Although I thought I had a pretty broad view of collaboration and interdisciplinary work, it's mind boggling how our languages and our cultures and our ways of doing things actually impede [our] goals (Duffy, 2002).

Ross Baker, University of Toronto, echoed this point and also noted the divide across competencies:

> One of the difficulties we face is that there are silos around the content...the informatics people talk to each other and the quality improvement/patient safety people talk to each other and the team people talk to each other and the evidence-based health care people talk to each other. And we need to be drawing the links more strongly...to think about ways to make linkages between those communities, the scholars, and the practitioners in order to try and identify ways in which they can learn from each other (Baker, 2002).

Creating a common language is no small task. Developing and adhering to distinct profession-specific terms may be a manifestation of professionals' desire to preserve identity, status, or control. This observation may explain, in part, why the competency movement in education, which has been gaining steam, has been contained within each profession, although spanning the continuum of a given profession also has proven difficult.

Some analysts characterize this movement toward competencies as a major paradigm shift and revolution for the 21st century (Carraccio et al., 2002; Lenburg, 1999). The competency movement actually began to gain some steam in the 1970s as a "back to basics" response to the more open-ended curricula of the 1960s that deemphasized basic skills. Innovative health professions schools of that era sought to integrate competencies into their curricula, but despite predictions that this was an idea whose time had come, competency-based education did not catch on. This may be because education leaders did not agree on a common set of competencies and ways to measure those competencies, nor did accreditors require such an approach (Carraccio et al., 2002; Luttrell et al., 1999).

A review of the literature suggests the close connection between common language and common competencies. For example, a group of 200 oversight and education professionals from 25 countries brought together to discuss systems for ensuring the competency of physicians noted the pressing need for common terminology to fulfill its charge (Bashook and Parboosingh, 1998). A recent review of attempts to incorporate competency-based training and evaluation in health professions education likewise stresses the importance of a common language (Carraccio et al., 2002; Parboosingh, 2000). Although the Europeans have been successful in defining a set of core competencies for physicians (Harden, 2002), a review of such efforts on the international front reveals a lack of standardized terminology and "wide variation…in the extent to which true competency-based learning objectives were instituted" (Carraccio et al., 2002:365). Box 6-1 describes one example of a successful interdisciplinary effort to define core competencies.

The committee believes that an interdisciplinary group, created under the auspices of the Department of Health and Human Services, should be charged with developing a common language across the health disciplines with the purpose of defining a core set of competencies and achieving threshold consensus around this core set. A similar notion was embraced by a participants in a summit working group focused on common language (see Appendix B).

Recommendation 1: DHHS and leading foundations should support an interdisciplinary effort focused on developing a common language, with the ultimate aim of achieving consensus across the health professions on a core set of competencies that includes patient-centered care, interdisciplinary teams, evidence-based practice, quality improvement, and informatics.

Box 6-1. Interdisciplinary Effort in Genetics Competencies

To date, efforts to move toward competency-based education have been made largely within the bounds of a given profession. An exception is an interdisciplinary effort, spearheaded by the **National Coalition for Health Professions Education in Genetics**, that involves the American Nurses Association, the American Medical Association, the National Human Genome Research Institute, and close to 100 other organizations. This collaborative effort has resulted in the development of core competencies for genetics education by the umbrella group.

Source: Reynolds (2000).

Integrating Competencies into Oversight Processes

The current call for oversight organizations to integrate competencies into their processes is in response to growing concerns about patient safety (Institute of Medicine, 2000; National Institutes of Health, 2002) the astounding geographic variation that exists in patient care that is not related to patient characteristics (O'Connor et al., 1996), and the associated desire on the part of public payers and consumers for increased accountability (Leach, 2002; Lenburg et al., 1999). In Europe, there also appears to be a sense that increased globalization will afford greater interaction among clinicians of different countries, generating the need for a set of core competencies that define clinicians regardless of where they are trained, and a related need for enhanced accountability (Harden, 2002). Box 6-2 describes one example of an effort to shift to a competency-based curriculum, in this case for pharmacy education.

During the last decade, competencies have begun to redefine the way some oversight organizations and professionals approach accreditation, as discussed in Chapter 5. In 1997, the American Council on Pharmaceutical Education (ACPE) adopted accreditation standards focused on 18 professional competencies (American Council on Pharmaceutical Education, 2002). In 1999, the Accreditation Council for Graduate Medical

---

Box 6-2. Large-Scale Reform in Pharmacy Education:

McWhorter as a Case Example

In 1997, the **American Council on Pharmaceutical Education** recommended that all pharmacy programs transition from a bachelor of pharmacy degree to an entry-level doctor of pharmacy program by the year 2000. Revising curricula and programs to satisfy this new paradigm was challenging, as schools learned that just taking their existing bachelors-level curriculum, adding a few things to it, and rearranging it a bit was not sufficient for making such a transition. Some schools embarked on a massive redesign of their programs. One, the **McWhorter School of Pharmacy at Samford University,** Birmingham, Alabama, developed its new curriculum using cross-functional teams of several faculty trained in quality improvement problem-solving skills and planning techniques. Using the Hoshin method (see Appendix C), the faculty collectively generated 23 competencies needed by its students and then redesigned the curriculum based on the defined competencies.

This competency-based curriculum stimulated the move from traditional, didactic lectures to teaching methods such as active learning and problem-based learning that necessitated much greater interaction between faculty and students, with a heavy emphasis on student learning groups providing systematic feedback to faculty. This reform of educational methods led to the redesign of the physical environment of the school to support these new interactive teaching methods, with a shift from fixed to movable seating, new construction of team meeting rooms, and roving microphones and electronic meeting tools for the classrooms. Today, the new curriculum emphasizes the need to readily access drug information by means of two core courses and a required advanced practice clerkship in drug information that serves as the training ground for students in the use of electronic tools, such as handheld personal digital assistants (PDAs).

Source: Armstrong and Barron (2002)

Education (ACGME) and the American Board of Medical Specialties (ABMS) endorsed six general competencies as the foundation for all graduate medical education; these competencies are currently being phased in (Accreditation Council for Graduate Medical Education, 2002). Until they have been fully implemented and evaluated, it remains to be seen what effect they will have on pharmacy and medical education, but they do overlap with the core competencies defined by the committee. In nursing, the two accrediting organizations also have defined competencies—which do not fully overlap with the core competencies defined here—but they differ in whether they require demonstration of such competencies (Commission on Collegiate Nursing Education, 2002; National League for Nursing Accrediting Commission, 1999). Finally, the curricula for the selected allied health professions examined in this report vary in the extent to which they incorporate the five competencies outlined herein (Collier, 2002).

The competency movement, however, does not have as much of a foothold in processes related to initial licensure or certification. As discussed in Chapter 5, requirements for maintaining license to practice vary considerably across the professions, as do requirements for those who pursue recognition or certification of clinical excellence. Further, research has raised serious questions about the efficacy of continuing education courses, the most common requirement for demonstrating ongoing competency (Davis et al., 1999; O'Brien et al., 2001; O'Brien et al., 2001). Some organizations, including the ABMS, the American Nurses Association, and the National Council of State Boards of Nursing, among others, have responded to these issues by taking steps to provide a better assessment of competency (Bashook et al., 2000; Whittaker et al., 2000).

Despite this increased momentum, one review found scarce evidence to support the efficacy of competency-based education (Carraccio et al., 2002). Yet the evidence that does exist demonstrates that competency- or outcome-based educational approaches lead to

improvements, such as better performance in licensing exams. Also, ways to assess competency are under development, and there does not yet appear to be a consensus on an appropriate approach. For example, some instruments are directly linked to particular definitions of competency (Chen et al., 1999), while others are more open-ended and attempt to assess aspects of competency that are difficult to define, such as management of ambiguity, professionalism, and teamwork (Epstein and Hundert, 2002).

Efforts to incorporate a core set of competencies across the professions into the full oversight framework—accreditation, licensing, and certification—would need to occur on the national, state, and local levels; coordinate both public- and private-sector oversight groups; and solicit input from professional associations and educational institutions. In developing a proposed strategy focused on oversight organizations, summit participants suggested a "big tent" approach (see Appendix C).

The committee believes that the involvement and support of DHHS, and specifically the Health Resources and Services Administration, would be important in getting this effort off the ground, in helping to establish a process for soliciting input from professional associations and the education community, and in identifying linkages and synergies from various oversight groups within and across professions. It is imperative to have such linkages among accreditation, licensure, and certification; it would mean very little, for example, if accreditation organizations required certain competencies, but these competencies were not reflected in licensing exams or requirements for continued practice. All processes must be linked so they are focused on the same outcome: enhancing the quality of patient care.

Recommendation 2: DHHS should provide a forum and support for a series of meetings involving the spectrum of oversight organizations across and within

the disciplines. Participants in these meetings would be charged with developing strategies for incorporating a core set of competencies into oversight activities, based on definitions shared across the professions. These meetings would actively solicit the input of health professions associations and the education community.

Strategies for incorporating the competencies into oversight processes would naturally differ across the oversight framework based on history, oversight approach, and structure, with consideration given to what steps particular groups have already taken. In all cases, the oversight bodies should proceed with deliberation. Efforts should be made to solicit comments on draft language related to new requirements, and to test new requirements wherever possible before implementation, such as through the use of provisional standards. Processes should also be established to monitor and evaluate new requirements to ensure that they are useful and not overly burdensome.

The experiences of ACPE and ACGME provide some guidance on how accrediting bodies, which operate at the national level, could incorporate competencies into their processes. Both ACPE and ACGME undertook an intensive, decade-long process of rethinking how they were preparing professionals for practice. They concluded, as did many reports that preceded their efforts, that fundamental change was necessary, and that they needed to move away from approaches that had become increasingly precise, prescriptive, and burdensome (Byrd, 2002).

What has not yet occurred is coordination across accrediting bodies of the various professions in defining a core set of competencies and designing related standards and measures. Such coordination could obviate the need for each accrediting body to reinvent the wheel, and synergies would likely result, enabling better communication and working relationships, as well as more consistent integration of the core competencies across

schools. This sort of coordinated effort would also help to ensure that educational innovators would not be stifled by outdated accreditation requirements. Organizational accreditors—such as the Joint Commission on Accreditation of Healthcare Organizations (JCAHO) and the National Committee for Quality Assurance (NCQA)—should likewise consider more fully how clinicians maintain competency in the core set of competencies outlined in this report.

Recommendation 3: Building upon previous efforts, accreditation bodies should move forward expeditiously to revise their standards so that programs are required to demonstrate—through process and outcome measures—that they educate students in both academic and continuing education programs in how to deliver patient care using a core set of competencies. In so doing, these bodies should coordinate their efforts.

As noted in Chapter 5, with the exception of patient-centered care, which is consistently included in examinations across the professions, licensing exams for health professionals vary considerably in whether they test for competency in the five core areas highlighted in this report (National Association of Boards of Pharmacy, 2002; National Council of State Boards of Nursing, 2001; United States Medical Licensing Exam, 2002). This situation also needs to be addressed and could be the focus of a subset of the oversight organizations described in recommendation 2.

In addition, separate, exclusive, and sometimes conflicting scope-of-practice acts and geographic restrictions on licensure need to be examined to determine whether they are a serious barrier to the full integration of competencies into practice. If so, consideration should be given to how they might be modified so that all clinicians can practice to the fullest extent of their technical training and ability, as well as take full advantage of new technologies, such as telemedicine (Safriet, 2002). While such an examination is beyond the scope of this report, the committee views it as important because of the influence scope of practice has on how clinicians are deployed and, in turn, how they are prepared for practice.

Finally, the committee believes that there should be an effort to integrate a core set of competencies into oversight processes focused on the continued competency of practicing clinicians. Such an effort would require coordination among an array of public- and private-sector licensing and certification organizations, within which there is currently little uniformity in approach across the professions or within a given profession across the states.

To begin with, state legislatures would need to require state licensing boards to insist that their licensees demonstrate competence to maintain their authority to practice. To date, state legislators have not insisted upon such a requirement, in part because there is disagreement about what constitutes evidence of competency and how often it should be demonstrated, not to mention who should judge such ability. Absent such a requirement, there will continue to be many boards that require only a fee for license renewal (Swankin, 2002) and many others that view continuing education as evidence of competence, even though such a linkage has not been demonstrated (O'Brien et al., 2001). Licensing boards also would need to consider clinician competency at varying career stages. For example, a veteran intensive care nurse or physician subspecialist should be expected to have a higher level of competence than a new graduate in either profession.

The committee believes that all health professions boards need to require demonstration of continued competency, and that they should move toward requiring rigorous tests for this purpose. Beyond licensing examinations, there is evidence to suggest that structured direct observations using standardized patients, peer assessments, and case- and essay-based questions are reliable ways to assess competency (Epstein and Hundert, 2002; Murray et al., 2000).

Recommendation 4: All health professions boards should move toward requiring licensed health professionals to demonstrate periodically their ability to deliver patient care—as defined by the five competencies identified by the committee—through direct measures of technical competence, patient assessment, evaluation of patient outcomes, and other evidence-based assessment methods. These boards should simultaneously evaluate the different assessment methods.

There is more uniformity among certifying organizations as compared with professional boards, in that nearly all require some means of demonstrating continuing competence. The vast majority allow for two or more approaches, and many also consider competency at various career stages. Moreover, in response to the paucity of evidence that taking continuing education courses improves practice outcomes, some certifying organizations are beginning to emphasize alternative measures that are more evidence based (American Board of Medical Specialties, 2000; American Nurses Association/NursingWorld.Org, 2001; Bashook et al., 2000; Board of Pharmaceutical Specialties, 2002; Federation of State Medical Boards, 2002; Finocchio et al., 1998; National Council of State Boards of Nursing, 1997-2000; Swankin, 2002a). Although such efforts are challenging to implement and often costly, certification bodies should only recognize continuing education courses as a valid method of maintaining competence if there is an evidence-based assessment of such courses; if clinicians select courses based on an assessment of their individual skills and knowledge; and if clinicians then demonstrate, through testing or other methods, that they have learned the course content.

The committee recognizes that there is a monetary and human resource cost to moving to evidence-based assessment, whether it is related to licensure or credentialing. Consequently, such assessments may need to be phased in, competency by competency, or less costly assessment methods identified. The committee also recognizes that increased investment in computer-based clinical records would provide the kind of rich clinical data necessary to fully realize competency-based licensure and certification.

Recommendation 5: Certification bodies should require their certificate holders to maintain their competence throughout the course of their careers by periodically demonstrating their ability to deliver patient care that reflects the five competencies, among other requirements.

Training Environments

Education does not occur in a vacuum; indeed, much of what is taught during the educational experience—and much of what is learned—lies outside formal academic coursework. This "hidden curriculum" of observed faculty or clinician behavior, informal interactions and conversations with fellow students and with faculty and practicing professionals, and the overall norms and culture of the training or practice environment is extremely powerful in shaping the values and attitudes of future health professionals (Ferrill et al., 1999; Hafferty and Franks, 1994; Maudsley, 2001).

What is learned through this hidden curriculum often can contradict the goals and content of the coursework that is formally offered. Courses may emphasize the importance of information technology in clinical care, but that message is not reinforced if students continue their education in health care organizations that are not equipped with information technology or whose faculty are not prepared to utilize informatics themselves. Students educated in a culture where the dominant belief is that physicians are all-knowing will likely not value shared decision making with patients regardless of whether they are taught to do so. Students educated in a

discontinuous system in which patients are quickly handed off to personnel in new venues of care will likely develop a narrow, task-specific view of illness, rather than a perspective of the whole patient or a systems orientation (Glick and Moore, 2001). Environments that punish those who make medical errors, with health providers blaming themselves, each other, or the patient, do not encourage students to explore alternative solutions, take risks, or apply quality improvement strategies to reduce future errors. In many training settings, the institutional norms are such that authoritarianism, boundaries of practice, and silos among professional disciplines are strictly enforced, and further reinforced by payment systems. In such settings, the value of interdisciplinary teams will likely not be grasped by students.

Role models, whether they be faculty, residents, clinician teachers, or other practicing health professionals, have a large part to play in this cultural influence. Branch (2000) documents the extent of the problem in medical education, with one survey of medical students showing that the majority believe their moral values were eroded during their clinical training. Another study showed widespread abuse of medical students by those in positions of power, and in one survey, 74 percent of residents reported directly observing mistreatment of patients. Equally alarming are studies demonstrating medical students' and residents' ambivalence and even antipathy toward management of the chronically ill as their education progresses (Davis et al., 2001). There is a need for health professions faculty to consider how they influence students' and residents' moral, ethical, and professional development as they become health practitioners, but little reform has been attempted in the area of faculty development and role modeling (Branch, 2000; Burack et al., 1999; Dechairo-Marino et al., 2001; Hundert et al., 1996; Maudsley, 2001). Summit panelist Bob Berenson, AcademyHealth, noted:

> I guess I'd go back to my days as a medical student and house officer... a lot of what I did back then was seeing role models, emulating what senior people were doing, what the faculty were doing ... And if the system gives incentives to not participate in multidisciplinary teams, that's what I'm going to learn even if somebody comes to a classroom and shows me a video of the potential benefits (Berenson, 2002).

The committee believes educational reform cannot happen without overall cultural reform. Panelist William Stead, Vanderbilt University, said at the summit:

> I think what we have to do is to require that our academic health-science centers become models of the type of clinical services that we want. I don't think we can expect people to learn to practice differently in a place that's run the old way (Stead, 2002).

The committee believes that initial support should be given to existing exemplary practice organizations including innovative academic health centers, that are already providing the interdisciplinary education and training necessary for staff to consistently deliver care that incorporates the core competencies. Further, the committee believes that these leading organizations should be identified as training models for other organizations, and should be given the resources necessary to test alternative approaches to providing curricula that integrate the core competencies. Such organizations should be encouraged to expand their efforts by opening their doors to other students, faculty, and clinicians. Emphasis should be given to all three populations, although approaches will differ depending upon which is targeted at any given time. In light of the evidence that faculty shortages and lack of preparedness are barriers to integrating the core competencies (Griner and Danoff, 2000; Halpern et al., 2001; Weed and Weed, 1999), faculty development should be a key focus of such centers. Summit participants also echoed the importance of faculty development (see Appendix C).

These exemplary organizations should serve as models for other practice and educational institutions as they seek to incorporate the core competencies into their curricula. They can help answer key operational questions, such as whether problem-based learning is the best approach to teaching these competencies, or other approaches would be preferable; which of these competencies might be taught by interdisciplinary teams in mixed settings and which discipline-by-discipline; and in terms of staging, when these competencies should be taught to students. These learning centers

---

Box 6-3 Faculty Development Programs

Faculty development programs, which are largely voluntary, operate at the institutional, regional, and national levels and employ varying approaches. Few appear to be interdisciplinary; in fact, there is a shortage of faculty able to teach the skills necessary to foster teamwork and collaboration, including negotiation, problem solving, and joint decision making (American Association of Colleges of Nursing, 1995; Hall and Weaver, 2001).

One new program—currently in the planning and prototype phase and bringing together health professions education organizations from eight disciplines and the Association of Academic Health Centers—is intended to be Web-based and is focused on developing teaching excellence and promoting the scholarship of teaching. The developers hope that this program—Health Professions Education Scholar—will become a key faculty development program that spans disciplines and is available to the full range of educational institutions (Meyer, 2002).

should also consider how to develop a sustainable business model, so that after an initial investment they could become self-sustaining in 3–5 years. Such a model might include provision of health care services or require training of outside clinicians and faculty.

There is precedence for focusing on learning centers that span occupations. For example, in health care there are examples of area health education centers that train a broad range of professionals with support from HRSA, while in other sectors, such as the airline industry, there are more comprehensive training efforts (O'Neil and the Pew Health Professions Commission, 1998). These learning organizations could provide centralized locations for information technology infrastructure, which would be an efficient way of aggregating costs across many organizations. Examples of the kinds of information technology that could be housed by these organizations include patient simulators and decision support tools incorporating electronic patient records and access to clinical databases.

Recommendation 6: Foundations, with support from education and practice organizations, should take the lead in developing and funding regional demonstration learning centers, representing partnerships between practice and education. These centers should leverage existing innovative organizations and be state-of-the art training settings focused on teaching and assessing the five core competencies.

There are many barriers to incorporating the five competencies into the practice environment, where medical residents and new graduates in nursing, pharmacy, and allied health obtain initial real-life training that leaves an important imprint on their future practice. Further, studies have shown that if there is too much of a disconnect between what is learned in school and the initial practice norms encountered, new graduates and residents become disheartened and cynical (Davis et al., 2001). In addition to the barriers of time constraints, oversight restrictions, resistance from the professions, and absence of political

---

Box 6-4 Refocusing on Teaching: Mayo Medical School

A common problem at teaching hospitals is clinicians being torn between their clinical care/revenue-generating responsibilities and their teaching responsibilities. Responding to this issue, **Mayo Medical School** began in the mid-1990s to make a systematic effort to develop and sustain a core faculty dedicated to innovation and excellence in education. The school decided to train a cadre of self-identified professionals as education experts as part of a core faculty program. A series of faculty development workshops addressed such topics as writing examinations, leading small-group discussions, and developing learning assessment cases. Each competency-based workshop has a structured curriculum with defined learning outcomes for learners. Courses are assessed and revised on the basis of student satisfaction and assessment.

The school also mapped out faculty career paths and made them as transparent as possible, organizing them into five career phases—early, midcareer, additional midcareer, senior, and leadership faculty—with increasing responsibilities and rewards. Recognizing that adult education principles are universal and apply to all health disciplines, the school plans to make the program interdisciplinary by targeting faculty involved in education at all levels within the institution in allied health, nursing, and medical residency education.

Source: Armstrong and Barron (2002).

will, the literature suggests, and the committee concurs, that the overall health care financing system is a large impediment to integrating the core competencies into practice. Therefore, the committee believes steps must be taken to explore alternative ways of paying clinicians so as to foster such integration.

The lack of a supportive financial structure becomes abundantly clear when one considers, for example, the kinds of services from which the chronically ill elderly would benefit and what Medicare fee-for-service will actually pay for. In the nation's most innovative practices, patients with, for example, diabetes and heart disease benefit greatly from patient education that helps them understand their conditions; how to manage them; and what changes are needed in diet, exercise, and tobacco and/or alcohol use. This education is provided and reinforced by a clinical team that includes a nurse practitioner, dietician, physician, and pharmacist, as well as follow-up group sessions with patients who have similar conditions that necessitate behavioral changes. Such patients appreciate the convenience of using a computer and at-home monitoring device to check blood sugar levels and blood pressure, as well as to transmit pictures of their hands and feet, as is currently the case for 1,500 patients in a Medicare demonstration in New York (IDEATel, 2002). Such patients also value having ready access to their clinicians via alternatives to office visits, such as e-mail or telephone, where appropriate. In these innovative care delivery systems, such patients also have ready access to needed drug therapies.

Currently, Medicare fee-for-service does not generally pay for clinician time spent providing education that enables such patients to make necessary lifestyle and behavioral changes, or for time spent helping patients help themselves by teaching them how to manage their condition actively with the support of technology. Medicare fee-for-service also does not pay for the work involved in coordinating and integrating these various patient services across teams and settings (Institute of Medicine, 2002). This is the case despite evidence showing that patients who are actively involved in managing and making decisions about their care have better quality and functional status outcomes at lower cost (Gifford et al., 1998; Johnson and Bootman, 1997; Superio-Cabuslay et al., 1996; Von Korff et al., 1998; Wagner et al., 2001).

As the largest payer, Medicare has a major effect on the system when it innovates (Institute of Medicine, 2002). And innovative government programs, such as the Program of All-Inclusive for the Elderly (PACE) (Centers for Medicaid and Medicare Services, 2002), have shown that changes in financing can foster redesign of care delivery. Moreover, the committee believes that patients with chronic conditions—a sizable proportion of whom are covered by Medicare—would benefit greatly from integration of the five competencies into practice. The committee encourages other payers as well to support changes in practice that will enhance patient care outcomes and provide fertile training grounds for new clinicians and residents. There are a number of different options that could serve as models for these payment experiments, including capitation, bundled payments, bonuses, withholds, and various ways to share risk and responsibility between clinicians and payers (Bailit Health Purchasing, 2002; Cooksey et al., 2002).

Recommendation 7: Through Medicare demonstration projects, the Centers for Medicare and Medicaid Services (CMS) should take the lead in funding experiments that will enable and create incentives for health professionals to integrate interdisciplinary approaches into educational or practice settings, with the goal of providing a training ground for students and clinicians that incorporates the five core competencies.

Research and Information

Along with oversight changes, supportive training environments, and related changes in financing, evidence of the efficacy of an educational intervention can be a catalyst for change in clinical education. However, evidence related to the link between health professions education and health care quality is not well developed, nor is there much evidence about various teaching approaches. And although there is significant public funding of health professions education, limited public and private resources are available for research that could help in determining whether the dollars are being well spent (Jordan, 2000; Leach, 2002). In addition, much of the research that does exist is discipline-specific and therefore does not reflect the current practice environment, where professional roles and responsibilities increasingly overlap.

The reasons why the education-related evidence base is so sparse are many and varied. Among them are that there are few incentives (including monetary incentives) for developing such an evidence base in either practice or education settings; that terms are not universal (as discussed above), so that it is difficult to assess the evidence; that there may be a sizable time lag between an intervention and an outcome; and that linking skills to patient outcomes is difficult because there are many intervening variables (Belfield et al., 2001). Specifically, a review of 117 trials in continuing education revealed that fewer than 20 percent use health care outcomes as their measure of effectiveness (Davis, 2000). Similarly, a review of 2,000 papers on continuing education showed that only about 5 percent assessed the relationship between course content and clinical outcomes (Jordan, 2000).

The committee believes that a more developed evidence base, particularly one linked to patient outcomes, would help make the case to educational institutions, regulators, professional societies, and others that dictate and shape health professions education that the acquisition and application of these competencies is essential to the provision of patient-centered care in a 21st-century health system. Summit participants agreed, and proposed a strategy focused on evidence-based education and the core competencies (see Appendix C).

The case for curriculum reform needs to be sound to convince institutions to add new topics to an already overcrowded curriculum, to modify teaching methods to cover the new topics (e.g., conducting sessions at the bedside or using problem-based learning), and to make the considerable investment in associated new infrastructure (e.g., informatics)—or to convince oversight bodies to require them to do any of these things. One study notes that accreditation bodies are reluctant to take risks or make a shift in orientation until there has been extensive validation of new approaches (Gelmon, 1996).

The committee wishes to underscore that traditional curricula in the health professions also lack an evidence base, raising questions about maintaining the status quo. Traditional health professions education is heavily compartmentalized and focused on the learning of discrete subject matter and the diagnosis and treatment of separate problems or diseases (Glick and Moore, 2001). Students are often trained in knowledge apart from both skills and attitudes. Various courses are added to prerequisites, with each discipline developing its own course structure. The result is that basic science, behavioral science, and clinical disciplines train students independently, with little interaction. An assumption is made that students, through their own devices, will assimilate, retain, and integrate all these courses and thus become competent. However, such compartmentalization leaves students unable to integrate the information and breeds "algorithmic thinking" (Saba, 2000) that often leads them to separate the physical and the psychosocial (Enarson and Burg, 1992; Wass et al., 2001). Reformers stress the need for a curriculum designed from a systems view that merges meaning, context, and connectedness among all concepts and components (Saba, 2000).

133

In addition to developing a better evidence base related to the competencies, it is important to assess how such competencies are taught. Evidence suggests that the traditional methods and approaches for teaching students and practicing clinicians may not be effective. As van der Vleuten et al. (2000) note, teaching is dominated by intuition and tradition, which do not always hold up when submitted to empirical verification. Within many academic settings, patient care and research are held to more rigorous standards, with teaching being guided more by personal beliefs and opinions and less by scholarly inquiry, evidence, and professional standards (Mennin, 1998).

For example, studies have shown that lecture-based teaching of isolated components, the most common way of imparting information in the academic setting, fails in that it does not provide a way for students to integrate or apply knowledge (Wass et al., 2001). Other approaches, such as problem-based learning, appear to engender more self-directed learning and do a better job of providing students with a way to integrate what they have already learned, (Rideout et al., 2002; Juul-Dam et al., 2001; Mennin, 1998) although some critics question the rigor of such an approach. With problem-based learning, embraced by approximately 100 medical schools (MedCases, 2002), students work on problem-solving exercises in small groups, actively applying their knowledge in a meaningful context (The Commonwealth Fund, 2002). Another educational approach that allows students to apply academic knowledge to practice is service learning, in which academic coursework is integrated with relevant community service. This approach also exposes students to cultural diversity, helps develop values, and fosters inductive reasoning (Hales, 1997; Callister and Hobbins-Garbett, 2000; Davidson, 2002; Schamess et al., 2000).

In the continuing education arena, the education is mainly course-based, an approach that has not been found effective in imparting new knowledge to existing practitioners. There also is no consistent evidence that problem-based learning in continuing education is superior to other educational strategies (Smits et al., 2002).

The leaders of U.S. health professions education may learn from recent European initiatives to develop the evidence base for education. One outcome of these initiatives is best-evidence medical education, which operates on two levels:

- What is taught: Development of an evidence base related to key competencies required in the practice environment, focusing on their relationship to quality.

- How it is taught: Reform of educational methods and practices based on available evidence about what works, and further development of the evidence base on the effectiveness of educational interventions.

The committee believes the time has come to focus energy and resources on developing a more robust and compelling evidence base about what educational content matters for patient care and what works in teaching clinicians so that educators, payers, and regulators can assess objectively what needs to be emphasized in the health professions curricula and what should be eliminated. Specific research areas should include a focus on particular dimensions of patient-centered care and interdisciplinary teams and their link to patient health, as well as on comparison of traditional approaches to evidence-based education. The research should also span disciplines.

Recommendation 8: The Agency for Healthcare Research and Quality (AHRQ) and private foundations should support ongoing research projects addressing the five core competencies and their association with individual and population health, as well as research related to the link between the competencies and evidence-based education. Such projects should involve researchers across two or more disciplines.

The committee further believes that if the vision of health professions education articulated in this report is to become a reality, ongoing monitoring of the effort will be required, and education-related measures will eventually need to be incorporated into national and regional quality-reporting efforts. The committee views this approach, which may be characterized as relatively market oriented, as complementary to the oversight approach, but less well developed at present.

The lack of standardized information about the quality of clinical education makes the job of leaders seeking to reform education that much more difficult. This lack of standardized measures also sets clinical education apart from the broader health care quality movement, in which such measures have affected where health care organizations channel their resources. A ranking—for example, by NCQA regarding health plan quality or by *U.S. News and World Report* regarding hospitals—forces leaders to focus their attention on improving performance on a given set of comparable metrics (National Committee for Quality Assurance, 2002; U.S. News and World Report, 2002). The National Healthcare Quality Report Card, anticipated for release by the Agency for Healthcare Research and Quality in 2003 and annually thereafter, will likely serve to further standardize quality measurement across all health sectors and focus attention on the strengths and weaknesses of the current system.

Yet no education-related measures are anticipated for inclusion in this first annual report (Agency for Health Care Research Quality, 2002). Such information might drive clinicians to improve and patients to demand improvement (Galvin, 2002; Institute of Medicine, 2002). While the committee acknowledges that there is still limited evidence about the link between health professionals' competencies and quality, a focused effort to develop education-related measures must begin now, given the amount of time required to develop and test prospective measures before they can be incorporated into report cards. The committee recognizes that initially there will be a small number of measures ready for public reporting.

Recommendation 9: AHRQ should work with a representative group of health care leaders to develop measures reflecting the core set of competencies, set national goals for improvement, and issue a report to the public evaluating progress toward these goals. AHRQ should issue the first report, focused on clinical educational institutions, in 2005 and produce annual reports thereafter.

Providing Leadership

Significant reform in health professions education is a challenge to say the least. The oversight framework is a morass of different organizations with differing requirements and philosophies, now under considerable pressure to demonstrate greater accountability (Batalden et al., 2002; O'Neil and the Pew Health Professions Commission, 1998). In academia, deans, department chairs, residency directors, and other leaders face a stream of requests for adding new elements to a curriculum that is already overcrowded. Shortages of key professionals, such as nurses and pharmacists, are another significant challenge. Moreover, funding for some academic health centers has been under pressure, and states are facing budget shortfalls that are causing them to trim education budgets, including funding for universities and community colleges (Griner and Blumenthal, 1998). In most academic health centers, education has become secondary to the operational needs of the institution's research and clinical missions (Enarson and Burg, 1992), with little reward provided for teaching (Cantor et al., 1993).

When change happens in health professions education, it does not happen overnight. Multiyear processes are required to develop, review, and achieve consensus on new requirements or methods before they can be implemented (Batalden et al., 2002). For example, to implement new accreditation

---

Box 6-5 Leadership and the Professions.

One recent important effort is the Charter on Medical Professionalism, which sets forth three principles and a set of 10 responsibilities to which all medical professionals should aspire regardless of their cultural background and where they practice across the globe. A project of the **ABIM Foundation, the American College of Physicians–American Society of Internal Medicine Foundation, and the European Federation of Internal Medicine**, this charter is intended to renew a sense of professionalism and support physicians' commitment to the primacy of patient welfare, patient autonomy, and social justice. The charter overlaps with many of the core competencies set forth in this report, including the primacy of patient welfare, a commitment to improving quality of care, and a commitment to scientific knowledge, among other responsibilities.

Source: ABIM Foundation (2002)

---

standards, accreditors need to go through a lengthy process of development that may take 2 years or longer and requires substantive input and discussion. The standards must be tested to see whether they achieve the stated objective (Gelmon, 1996). Once the standards have been finalized, they must be phased in over a 3-year period or longer. Within institutions, changing course requirements in response to new accreditation requirements may take many years, and often involves a highly charged political conflict within and across departments and disciplines.

Given this environment, the committee believes that reform of health professions education will be possible only through the skill and dedication of a broad set of health care leaders from the professions, educational institutions, and oversight bodies, among others. A review of the literature underscores the importance of leadership. One analysis and synthesis of 44 curriculum reform efforts revealed that leadership is the factor most often cited as affecting the success of such efforts (Bland et al., 2000). The authors also note the importance of five other factors critical to curriculum change—a cooperative climate, participation by organization members, human resource development, a manageable political environment, and ongoing evaluation of the effort—and conclude that leadership is the pivotal element in success, as leaders control or substantially influence all the other factors (Bland et al., 2000). Other studies also confirm

the centrality of leadership (Mennin, 1998). Box 6-6 describes some noteworthy examples of interdisciplinary leadership.

Consequently, the committee believes that to maintain momentum for reform in clinical education, there will need to be biennial summits at which leaders who have demonstrated a real commitment to implementing the committee's overarching vision can gather. These summits should serve as a forum for taking stock—including reviewing education-related performance measures and, over time, related trends against goals—and defining future plans. There should be a written report issued from the summit that captures such information and communicates it more broadly to the field.

Recommendation 10: Beginning in 2004, a biennial interdisciplinary summit should be held involving health care leaders in education, oversight processes, practice, and other areas. This summit should focus on both reviewing progress against explicit targets and setting goals for the next phase with regard to the five competencies and other areas necessary to prepare professionals for the 21st-century health system.

Box 6-6. Noteworthy Interdisciplinary Leadership Efforts

The **National Center for Health Care Leadership (NCHCL),** a nonprofit organization, is focused on the initial and ongoing education of health care managers. It collaborates with established educational and professional organizations, and its efforts involve a broad cross section of health professionals. The organization's goals include establishing core competencies for health care managers at all career stages and defining protocols for their continuous learning. The board of NCHCL consists of practitioners, educators, and researchers (National Center for Healthcare Leadership, 2002).

The **Centre for the Advancement of Interprofessional Education** in the United Kingdom draws its members from the fields of medicine, nursing, allied health, social work, and management. The organization's charge is to promote interprofessional education, focused on discrete, vulnerable populations, so that the care for these groups will be better integrated and coordinated across the professions and between health care and social service organizations. Education leaders from these disciplines are brought together and asked to lead the charge for educational reform as it relates to a particular population (Horder, 2000).

The **Partnership for Quality Education**, a nonprofit organization supported by foundations, seeks to bring about change in primary care education by supporting partnerships among medical residency programs, nurse practitioner programs, and managed care organizations. In some cases, schools of social work and pharmacy also are involved in the partnerships, which focus on better preparing professionals to manage the quality and cost of care through collaborative practices and interdisciplinary teams (Partnership for Quality, 2002).

Conclusion

The committee has set forth 10 major recommendations for reforming health professions education to enhance quality and meet the evolving needs of patients. Each of these recommendations focuses on ways of integrating a core set of competencies into health professions education. Taken together, they represent a mix of approaches related to oversight processes, the practice environment, research, public reporting, and leadership.

The staging of these recommendations is important. The first step is to articulate common terms so that shared definitions can inform interdisciplinary discussions about core competencies. Once the disciplines have agreed on a core set of competencies, public and private oversight bodies can consider how to incorporate such competencies into their processes—providing a catalyst for many

educational institutions and professional associations, as well as support for those who have already moved toward adopting a competency-based approach. The committee believes that the development of common language and definition of core competencies should happen as rapidly as possible and by no later than 2004, given that the integration of core competencies into oversight processes will take considerable time, perhaps a decade or more if the efforts of ACGME and ACPE are any guide.

As the work of integrating core competencies into oversight processes proceeds, the efforts of leading practice and education organizations to provide a training environment that integrates the core competencies into care delivery should be fostered through regional demonstration learning centers and Medicare demonstration projects. Simultaneously with these efforts, AHRQ and private foundations

---

should provide support for research focused on the efficacy of the competencies and competency education and, most important, develop a set of measures reflecting the core set of competencies, along with national goals for improvement. Given that the committee calls upon AHRQ to issue a first report on health professions educational institutions by 2005, albeit with a limited number of initial measures, efforts related to reporting must begin immediately. Finally, the committee believes that biennial summits of health care leaders who control and shape education—starting in 2004—will be an important mechanism for integrating and furthering the efforts of those developing measures, practice and education innovators, researchers, and leaders from oversight organizations.

The committee is confident that its recommendations are both sound and feasible to implement because they are supported by a literature review, and informed by a broad range of leaders who shape education both directly and indirectly. Building a bridge to cross the quality chasm in health care cannot be done in isolation. The committee hopes that this report will jump start other efforts to reform clinical education, both individually and collectively, so that it focuses on continually reducing the burden of illness, injury, and disability, with the ultimate aim of improving the health status, functioning, and satisfaction of the American people (President's Advisory Commission on Consumer Protection and Quality in the Health Care Industry, 1998). The public deserves nothing less.

References

ABIM Foundation. 2002. Medical professionalism in the new millennium: A physician charter. *Annals of Internal Medicine* 136 (3):243-46.

Accreditation Council for Graduate Medical Education. 2002. "ACGME Outcome Project." Online. Available at http://www.acgme.org/outcome/about/faq.asp [accessed Aug. 27, 2002].

Agency for Healthcare Research and Quality. 2002. "NHQR Preliminary Measure Set." Online. Available at http://www.ahrq.gov/qual/nhqr02/nhqrprelim.htm [accessed Fall, 2002].

American Association of Colleges of Nursing. 1995. *Interdisciplinary Education and Practice.* California: AACN.

American Board of Medical Specialties. 2000. "Recertification and Time-Limited Certification." Online. Available at http://www.abms.org/Downloads/General_Requirements/Table6.PDF [accessed Nov., 2002].

American Council on Pharmaceutical Education. 2002. "ACPE Web site." Online. Available at www.acpe.edu [accessed May 1, 2002].

American Nurses Association/NursingWorld.Org. 2001. "On-line Health and Safety Survey: Key Findings." Online. Available at http://nursingworld.org/surveys/keyfind.pdf [accessed 2002].

Armstrong, E.G., and J.W. Barron. 2002. Issues and Strategies for Reforming Professional Culture: Lessons from the Health Professions and Beyond. *IOM Commissioned Background Paper*

Bailit Health Purchasing. 2002. *Provider Incentive Models for Improving Quality of Care.* Washington, DC: National Health Care Purchasing Institute.

Baker, R. 2002. ""Crossing the Quality Chasm: Next Steps for Health Professions Education"; Panel Discussion." Online. Available at http://www.kaisernetwork.org/health_cast/hcast_index.cfm?display=detail&hc=601 [accessed Nov. 12, 2002].

Bashook, P.G., S.H. Miller, J. Parboosingh, and S.D. Horowitz. 2000. "Credentialing Physician Specialists: A World Perspective." Online. Available at http://www.abms.org/Downloads/Conferences/Credentialing%20Physician%20Specialists.pdf [accessed Sept. 15, 2002].

Bashook, P.G., and J. Parboosingh. 1998. Continuing medical education: Recertification and the maintenance of competence. *British Medical Journal* 316 (7130):545-48.

Batalden, P., D. Leach, S. Swing, H. Dreyfus, and S. Dreyfus. 2002. General competencies and accreditation in graduate medical education. *Health Affairs* 21 (5):103-11.

Belfield, C., H. Thomas, A. Bullock, R. Eynon, and D. Wall. 2001. Measuring effectiveness for best evidence medical education: A discussion. *Medical Teacher* 23 (2):164-70.

Berenson, B. 2002. ""Crossing the Quality Chasm: Next Steps for Health Professions Education"; Panel Discussion." Online. Available at http://www.kaisernetwork.org/health_cast/hcast_index.cfm?display=detail&hc=601 [accessed Nov. 12, 2002].

Bland, C.J., S. Starnaman, L. Wersal, L. Moorhead-Rosenberg, S. Zonia, and R. Henry. 2000. Curricular change in medical schools: How to succeed. *Academic Medicine* 75 (6):575-94.

Branch, W.T., Jr. 2000. Supporting the moral development of medical students. *Journal of General Internal Medicine* 15 (7):503-8.

Buckingham, C.D., and A. Adams. 2000. Classifying clinical decision making: A unifying approach. *Journal of Advanced Nursing* 32 (4):981-89.

Burack, J.H., D.M. Irby, J.D. Carline, R.K. Root, and E.B. Larson. 1999. Teaching compassion and respect: Attending physicians' responses to problematic behaviors. *Journal of General Internal Medicine* 14 (1):49-55.

Busari, J., A. Scherpbier, C. Van der Vleuten, and G. Essed. 2000. Residents perception of their role in teaching undergraduate students in the clinical setting. *Medical Teacher* 22 (4):348.

Byrd, G. 2002. Can the profession of pharmacy serve as a model for health informationist professionals? *Journal of Medical Library Association* 90 (1):68-75.

Callister, L.C., and D. Hobbins-Garbett. 2000. Enter to learn, go forth to serve: Service learning in nursing education. *Journal of Professional Nursing* 16 (3):177-83.

Cantor, J.C., L.C. Baker, and R.G. Hughes. 1993. Preparedness for practice. Young physicians views of their professional education. *JAMA* 270 (9):1035-40.

Carraccio, C., S.D. Wolfsthal, R. Englander, K. Ferentz, and C. Martin. 2002. Shifting paradigms: From flexner to competencies. *Academic Medicine* 77 (5):361-67.

Center for the Health Professions University of California San Francisco. 2002. "Leadership Initiative for Nursing Education (LINE)." Online. Available at http://www.futurehealth.ucsf.edu/line.html [accessed Nov., 2002].

Centers for Medicaid and Medicare Services. 2002. "Program of All Inclusive Care For the Elderly (PACE)." Online. Available at http://www.cms.hhs.gov/pace/ [accessed 2002].

Chen, S.P., N.E. Ervin, Y. Kim, and S.C. Vonderheid. 1999. Competency in community-oriented health care. Instrument development. *Evaluation and Health Professions* 22 (3):358-70.

Closs, S.J. and F.M. Cheater. 1999. Evidence for nursing practice: A clarification for the issues. *Journal of Advanced Nursing* 30 (1):10-17.

Collier, S. March 2002. Workforce Shortages. Personal communication to Ann Greiner.

Commission on Collegiate Nursing Education. 2002. "CCNE Accreditation." Online. Available at http://www.aacn.nche.edu/Accreditation/ [accessed 2002].

Cooksey, J.A., K.K. Knapp, S.M. Walton, and J.M. Cultice. 2002. Challenges to the pharmacist profession from escalating pharmaceutical demand. *Health Aff (Millwood)* 21 (5):182-88.

Davidson, R. 2002. Coummunity-based education and problem solving: The community health scholars program at University of Florida. *Teaching & Learning in Medicine* 14 (3):178.

Davis, B.E., D.B. Nelson, O.J. Sahler, F.A. McCurdy, R. Goldberg, and L.W. Greenberg. 2001. Do clerkship experiences affect medical students attitudes toward chronically ill patients? *Academic Medicine* 76 (8):815-20.

Davis, D. 2000. Clinical practice guidelines and the translation of knowledge: The science of continuing medical education. *Canadian Medical Association Journal:* 163 (10):1278-79.

Davis, D., M.A. OBrien, N. Freemantle, F.M. Wolf, P. Mazmanian, and A. Taylor-Vaisey. 1999. Impact of formal continuing medical education: Do conferences, workshops, rounds, and other traditional continuing education activities change physician behavior or health care outcomes? *Journal of American Medical Association* 282 (9):867-74.

Dechairo-Marino, A.E., M. Jordan-Marsh, G.

Traiger, and M. Saulo. 2001. Nurse/physician collaboration: Action research and the lessons learned. *Journal Nursing Administration* 31 (5):223-32.

Duffy, D. 2002. ""Crossing the Quality Chasm: Next Steps for Health Professions Education"; Panel Discussion." Online. Available at http://www. kaisernetwork.org/health_cast/hcast_index.cfm? display=detail&hc=601 [accessed Nov. 12, 2002].

Enarson, C., and F.D. Burg. 1992. An overview of reform initiatives in medical education. 1906 through 1992. [Review] [22 refs]. *Journal of American Medical Association* 268 (9):1141-43.

Epstein, R.M., and E.M. Hundert. 2002. Defining and assessing professional competence. *Journal of the American Medical Association* 287 (2):226-35.

Evers, G. 2001. Naming Nursing: Evidence-based nursing. *Nursing Diagnosis* 12 (4):137-42.

Federation of State Medical Boards. 1998. "Maintaining State-Based Medical Licensure and Discipline: A Blueprint for Uniform and Effective Regulation of the Medical Profession." Online. Available at http://www.fsmb.org/ uniform.htm [accessed Jan. 12, 2001].

Ferrill, M.J., L.L. Norton, and S.J. Blalock. 1999. Determining the statistical knowledge of pharmacy practitioners: A survey and review of the literature 1. *American Journal of Pharmaceutical Education* 63 (3)

Galvin, B. April 2002. Health Professions Education. Personal communication to IOM Committee.

Gelmon, S.B. 1996. Can educational accreditation drive interdisciplinary learning in the health professions? *Joint Commission Journal on Quality Improvement* 22 (3):213-22.

Gifford, A.L., D.D. Laurent, V.M. Gonzales, et al. 1998. Pilot randomized trial of education to improve self-management skills of men with symptomatic HIV/AIDS. *Journal of Acquired Immune Deficiency Syndromes and Human Retrovirology* 18 (2):136-44.

Glick, T.H., and G.T. Moore. 2001. Time to learn: The outlook for renewal of patient-centred education in the digital age. *Medical Education* 35 (5):505-9.

Griner, P.F.M., and D.M. Danoff. 2000. Sustaining change in medical education. *Journal of American Medical Association* 283 (18):2429-31.

Griner, P., and D. Blumenthal. 1998. New bottles for vintage wines: The changing management of the medical school faculty. *Academic Medicine* 73 (6):720-724.

Guyatt, G.H., R.B. Haynes, R.Z. Jaeschke, D.J. Cook, L. Green, C.D. Naylor, M. Wilson, and W.S. Richardson. 2000. Users guide to the medical literature: XXV. Evidence-based medicine: Principles for applying the users guides to patient care. *Journal of American Medical Association* 284 (10):1290-1296.

Hafferty, F.W., and R. Franks. 1994. The hidden curriculum, ethics teaching, and the structure of medical education. *Academic Medicine* 69 (11):861-71.

Hales, A.P.R. 1997. Service-learning within the nursing curriculum. *Nurse Educator* 22 (2):15-18.

Hall, P., and L. Weaver. 2001. Interdisciplinary education and teamwork: A long and winding road. *Medical Education* 35 (9):867-75.

Halpern, J. 1996. The measurement of quality of care in the veterans health administration. *Medical Care* 34 (3):55-68.

Halpern, R., M.Y. Lee, P.R. Boulter, and R.R. Phillips. 2001. A synthesis of nine major reports on physicians competencies for the emerging practice environment. *Academic Medicine* 76 (6):606-15.

Harden, R.M. 2002. Developments in outcome-based education. *Medical Teacher* 24 (2):117-20.

Harmening, D.M. 1999. "Pioneering Allied Health Clinical Education Reform. A National Consensus Conference." Online. Available at ftp://ftp.hrsa.gov/bhpr/publications/cerpdf.pdf [accessed Aug., 2002].

Health Resources and Services Administration. 1999. *Building the Future of Allied Health: Report of the Implementation Task Force of the National Commission on Allied Health.* Rockville, MD: Health Resources and Services Administration.

Higgs, J.P., A.M. Burn, and M.M. Jones. 2001.

Integrating clinical reasoning and evidence-based practice. *Association of Critical-Care Nurses Clinical Issues: Advanced Practice in Acute & Critical Care* 12 (4):482-90.

Horder, J. 2000. Leadership in a multiprofessional context. *Medical Education* 34:203-5.

Hundert, E.M., F. Hafferty, and D. Christakis. 1996. Characteristics of the informal curriculum and trainees ethical choices. *Academic Medicine* 71 (6):624-42.

IDEATel. "Informatics for Diabetes Education and Telemedicine." Online. Available at http://www.ideal.org/info.html [accessed Sept. 12, 2002].

Institute of Medicine. 2000. *To Err Is Human: Building a Safer Health System.* Linda T. Kohn, Janet M. Corrigan, and Molla S. Donaldson, eds. Washington, DC: National Academy Press.

———. 2001. *Crossing the Quality Chasm: A New Health System for the 21st Century.* Washington, DC: National Academy Press.

———. 2002. *Leadership By Example.* Washington, DC: National Academies Press.

Johnson, J.A., and J.L. Bootman. 1997. Drug-related morbidity and mortality and the economic impact of pharmaceutical care. *American Journal of Health-System Pharmacy* 54 (5):554-58.

Jordan, S. 2000. Educational input and patient outcomes: Exploring the gap. *Journal of Advanced Nursing* 31 (2):461-71.

Josiah Macy Jr. Foundation. 2002. "Leadership Training for Safety Net Hospitals." Online. Available at http://www.umassmed.edu/externalwindow.cfm?URL=http://www.josiahmacyfoundation.org/jmacy1.html&Link=http://www.umassmed.edu/macy/&DeptName=Macy%20Initiative%20in%20Health%20Communication [accessed Nov. 8, 2002].

Juul-Dam, N.M., S.M. Brunner, R.M. Katzenellenbogen, M.M. Silverstein, and D.A. M.M. Christakis. 2001. Does problem-based learning improve residents self-directed learning? *Archives of Pediatrics* 155 (6):673-75.

Lang, N.M. 1999. Discipline-based approaches to evidence-based practice: A view from nursing.

Joint Commission Journal on Quality Improvement 25 (10):539-44.

Lavin, M.A., I. Ruebling, R. Banks, L. Block, M. Counte, G. Furman, P. Miller, C. Reese, V. Viehmann, and J. Holt. 2001. Interdisciplinary health professional education: A historical review. *Advances in Health Sciences Education* 6 (1):25-47.

Leach, D.C. 2002. Competence is a habit. *Journal of the American Medical Association* 287 (2):243-44.

Lenburg, C. 1999. "Redesigning Expectations for Initial and Continuing Competence for Contemporary Nursing Practice." Online. Available at http://www.nursingworld.org/ojin/topic 10/tpc10_1.htm [accessed Aug. 19, 2002].

Lenburg, C., R. Redman, and P. Hinton. 1999. "Competency Assessment: Methods for Development and Implementation in Nursing Education." Online. Available at in cabinet [accessed Mar. 19, 2002].

Luttrell, M.F., C.B. Lenburg, J.C. Scherubel, S.R. Jacob, and R.W. Koch. 1999. Competency outcomes for learning and performance assessment. Redesigning a BSN curriculum. *Nursing Health Care Perspectives* 20 (3):134-41.

Marwick, C. 2000. Will evidence-based practice help span gulf between medicine and law? *Journal of American Medical Association* 283 (21):2775-76.

Masys, D.R., P.F. Brennan, J.G. Ozbolt, M. Corn, and E.H. Shortliffe. 2000. Are medical informatics and nursing informatics distinct disciplines? The 1999 ACMI debate. *Journal of American Medical Information Association* 7 (3):304-12.

Maudsley, R.F. 2001. Role models and the learning environment: Essential elements in effective medical education. *Academic Medicine* 76:432-34 .

Mazurek, B. 2002. Strategies for overcoming barriers in implementing evidence-based practice. *Periatric Nursing* 28 (2):159-61.

MedCases. 2002. "Forces For Medical Education Curriculum Reform." Online. Available at http://www.medcases.pdfs/pdf_page1.htm [accessed Oct. 27, 2002].

Mennin, S., and S.P. Kalishman. 1998. Issues and strategies for reform in medical education: Lessons from eight medical schools. *Academic Medicine (Supplement)* 73 (9)

Meyer, S. 19 December 2002. Health Professions Scholar. Personal communication to Ann Greiner.

Mitchell, G. 1999. Evidence-based practice: Critique and alternative view. *Nursing Science Quarterly* Vol. 12, No. 1:30-35.

Murray, E., L. Gruppen, P. Catton, R. Hays, and J.O. Woolliscroft. 2000. The accountability of clinical education: Its definition and assessment. *Medical Education* 34 (10):871-79.

National Association of Boards of Pharmacy. 2002. "Examinations -- NAPLEX." Online. Available at http://www.nabp.net/ [accessed Aug. 10, 2002].

National Center for Healthcare Leadership. 2002. "Strategic Plan." Online. Available at in cabinet [accessed Aug. 30, 2002].

National Committee for Quality Assurance. 2002. "What Does NCQA Review When It Accredits an HMO?" Online. Available at http://www. ncqa.org/Programs/Accreditation/MCO/ mcostdsoverview.htm [accessed 2002].

National Council of State Boards of Nursing. 2000. "Nurse Licensure Compact." Online. Available at http://www.ncsbn.org/public/ nurselicensurecompact/mutual_recognition.htm [accessed Aug., 2002].

————. 2001. "NCLEX - RN@ Examination: Test Plan for the National Council Licensure Examination for Registered Nurses." Online. Available at http://www.ncsbn.org/public/ testing/res/NCSBNRNTestPlanBooklet.pdf [accessed Aug., 2002].

National Institutes of Health. 2002. "National Institute of Health Web site." Online. Available at www.nih.gov [accessed May 13, 2002].

National League for Nursing Accrediting Commission. 1999. "1999 Standards and Criteria and Interpretative Guidelines." Online. Available at http://www.nlnac.org/Manual% 20&%20IG/01_accreditation_manual.htm [accessed Aug. 14, 2002].

OBrien, T., N. Freemantle, A.D. Oxman, F. Wolf, D. A. Davis, and J. Herrin. 2001. Continuing education meetings and workshops: Effects on professional practice and health care outcomes. *Cochrane Database System Review* (2): CD003030.

OConnor, G.T., S.K. Plume, E.M. Olmstead, J.R. Morton, C.T. Maloney, W.C. Nugent, F. Hernandez, Jr. , R. Clough, B.J. Leavitt, L.H. Coffin, C.A. Marrin, D. Wennberg, J.D. Birkmeyer, D.C. Charlesworth, D.J. Malenka, H.B. Quinton, and J.F. Kasper. 1996. A regional intervention to improve the hospital mortality associated with coronary artery bypass graft surgery. The Northern New England Cardiovascular Disease Study Group. *Journal of the American Medical Association* 275 (11):841-46.

ONeil, E. H. and the Pew Health Professions Commission. 1998. *Recreating health professional practice for a new century - The fourth report of the PEW health professions Commission.* San Francisco, CA: Pew Health Professions Commission.

Parboosingh, J. 2000. Credentialing physicians: Challenges for continuing medical education. *Journal of Continuing Education in the Health Professions* 20 p188 (3):3p.

Partnership for Quality. 2002. "About PQE." Online. Available at www.pqe.com [accessed 2002].

Pomeroy, W.M., and I. Philp. 1994. Healthcare teams: An interdisciplinary workshop for undergraduates. *Medical Teacher*:6p.

Prentice, T., and T. Bentley. 1999 . Counting on clinical terms: The Healthcare Intervention Aggregation project. *British Journal of Healthcare Computing & Information Management* 16(1):38-40.

President's Advisory Commission on Consumer Protection and Quality in the Health Care Industry. 1998. "Quality First: Better Health Care for All Americans." Online. Available at http://www.hcqualitycommission.gov/final/ [accessed Sept. 9, 2002].

Rideout, E., V. England-Oxford, B. Brown, F. Fothergill-Bourbonnais, C. Ingram, G. Benson, M. Ross, and A. Coates. 2002. A comparison of problem-based and conventional curricula in nursing education. *Advances in Health Sciences Education* 7:3-17.

Saba, G.W. 2000. Preparing healthcare

professionals for the 21st century: Lessons from chirons cave. *Families, Systems & Health: The Journal of Collaborative Family HealthCare* 18 (3):353-64.

Sackett, D. 1998. Finding and applying evidence during clinical rounds. *Journal of American Medical Association* 280 (15):1336-38.

Safriet, B. 2002. Closing the gap between can and may in health-care providers scopes of practices. *Yale Journal on Regulation* 19 (2):301-34.

Satya-Murti, S. 2000. Evidence-based clinical practice: Concepts and approaches. *The Journal of American Medical Association* 282 (17):2306-7.

Schamess, A., R. Wallis, R.D. David, and Eiche. 2000. Academic medicine, service learning, and the health of the poor. *American Behavioral Scientist* 43 (5):793-08.

Shaver, J. 24 September 2002. Personal Conversation . Personal communication to Ann Greiner.

Smits, P., J. Verbeek, and C. de Buisonje. 2002. Problem based learning in continuing medical education: A review of controlled evaluation studies. *British Medical Journal* 324 (7330)

Stead, W. 2002. "Crossing the Quality Chasm: Next Steps for Health Professions Education; Panel Discussion." Online. Available at http://www. kaisernetwork.org/health_cast/hcast_index.cfm? display=detail&hc=601 [accessed Nov. 12, 2002].

Superio-Cabuslay, E., M.M. Ward, and K.R. Lorig. 1996. Patient education interventions in osteoarthritis and rheumatoid arthritis: A meta-analytic comparison with nonsteroidal anti-inflammatory drug treatment. *Arthritis Care Research* 9 (4):292-301.

Swankin, D.S. 2002. *Results of a Survey of Selected State Health Licensing Boards and Health Voluntary Certification Agencies Concerning their Continuing Competence Programs and Requirements*. Washington, DC: Citizen Advocacy Center.

The Commonwealth Fund. 2002. *Training Tomorrows Doctors*. Boston, MA:

U.S. News and World Report. "Latest Hospital Rankings." Online. Available at www.usnews. com/usnews/nycu/health/hosptl/tophosp.htm

[accessed Summer, 2002].

United States Medical Licensing Exam. 2002. "United States Medical Licensing Examination - Steps 1, 2, 3." Online. Available at http://www. usmle.org/step1/intro.htm [accessed Aug. 10, 2002].

Von Korff, M., J.E. Moore, K.R. Lorig, et al. 1998. A randomized trial of a lay person-led self-management group intervention for back pain patients in primary care. *Spine* 23 (23):2608-51.

Wagner, E.H., R.E. Glasgow, C. Davis, A.E. Bonomi, L. Provost, D. McCulloch, P. Carver, and C. Sixta. 2001. Quality improvement in chronic illness care: A collaborative approach. *Joint Commission Journal on Quality Improvement* 27 (2):63-80.

Wass, V., C. Van der Vleuten, J. Shatzer, and R. Jones. 2001. Assessment of clinical competence. *Lancet* 357 (9260):945-49.

Weed, L.L. and L. Weed. 1999. Opening the black box of clinical judgment. Part II: consumer protection and the patients role. *British Medical Journal*. November 13

Welch, H.G., and J.D. Lurie. 2000. Teaching evidence-based medicine: Caveats and challenges. *Academic Medicine* 75 (3):235-40.

Whittaker, S., W. Carson, and M.C. Smolenski. 2000. Assuring continued competence -- policy questions and approaches: How should the profession respond? *Online Journal of Issues in Nursing*:18.

Woolf, S.H. 2000. Taking critical appraisal to extremes: The need for balance in the evaluation of evidence. *Journal of Family Practice* 49 (12):1081-85.

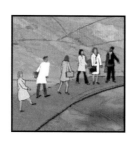

Appendix A
Committee Biographies

Edward M. Hundert, *Co-Chair,* has been President of Case Western Reserve University since August 2002. He was previously Dean of the School of Medicine and Dentistry and Professor of Psychiatry and Medical Humanities at the University of Rochester. For the 3 years before his appointment as Dean in 2000, Dr. Hundert was the University of Rochester's Senior Associate Dean for Medical Education. In that capacity, he led the effort of the medical school's faculty and students to create the Double Helix Curriculum—a sweeping integration of the basic and clinical sciences across the 4-year medical school experience. During the years before he came to Rochester, Dr. Hundert served as Associate Professor of Psychiatry and Associate Dean for Student Affairs at Harvard Medical School, as well as Assistant Director of Psychiatric Residency Training at McLean Hospital. He taught medical ethics and psychiatry in the curriculum, and was active in ethics as Chairman of the Ethics Committees of both McLean Hospital and the Massachusetts Psychiatric Society. His pioneering research on the informal curriculum in medical education helped shape the national discussion of professionalism in medicine. Dr. Hundert was voted the faculty member who did the most for the class by the Harvard Medical School graduating class for 6 successive years.

Mary Wakefield, *Co-Chair,* is Director, Center for Rural Health, at the University of North Dakota School of Medicine and Health Sciences. Previously, Dr. Wakefield served as Professor and Director of the Center for Health Policy and Ethics at George Mason University and as Chief of Staff for two United States Senators. During her tenure on Capitol Hill, she co-chaired the Senate Rural Health Caucus Staff Organization. In this capacity, she was directly involved with a wide range of rural health policy issues, including recruitment and retention of health care providers, reimbursement, emergency services, telemedicine, rural research, and interdisciplinary education. Dr. Wakefield serves on many health-related advisory boards, and in March 1997 was appointed to

President Clinton's Advisory Commission on Consumer Protection and Quality in the Health Care Industry. In 1999, Dr. Wakefield was appointed by the U.S. Comptroller General to a 3-year term on the Medicare Payment Advisory Commission, which is responsible for advising the U.S. Congress on the Medicare program. In June 1999, she was appointed to the Advisory Committee to the Office of Rural Health Policy, Department of Health and Human Services. Dr. Wakefield has previously served as a member of the Institute of Medicine's (IOM) technical panel on Communication of Quality of Care Information, the Committee on Quality of Health Care in America, and the subcommittees on Community Effects of Uninsured Populations and Building the 21st Century Health System.

J. Lyle Bootman is Dean and Professor of Pharmacy, Medicine, and Public Health at The University of Arizona College of Pharmacy. He is also the founder and Executive Director of The University of Arizona Center for Health Outcomes and PharmacoEconomic Research, one of the first such centers developed in the world. Dr. Bootman is a former President of the American Pharmaceutical Association. He has received numerous awards for outstanding scientific achievement, most notably from the American Association of Pharmaceutical Scientists and the American Pharmaceutical Association. He has also received the George Archambault Award, the highest honor given by the American Society of Consultant Pharmacists, and the Latiolais Honor Medal, the highest honor in managed health care. His research regarding the outcomes of drug-related morbidity and mortality receives worldwide attention by the professional and public media. He serves as an advisor to leading pharmaceutical companies, universities, and health care organizations throughout the world. In 1998, Dr. Bootman was elected to the IOM, where he currently serves on the Board of Health Care Services.

Christine K. Cassel (IOM) is Dean of the School of Medicine at Oregon Health and Science University. She is Chairman of the Henry L. Schwarz Department of Geriatrics and Adult Development and Professor of Geriatrics and Internal Medicine at the Mount Sinai Medical Center. She joined Mount Sinai in 1995 after 10 years as Chief of General Internal Medicine at the University of Chicago, where she was also Professor of Medicine and Public Policy Studies; Chief of the Section on General Internal Medicine; Director of the Center on Aging, Health, and Society; Director of the Center for Health Policy Research; and George M. Eisenberg Professor of Geriatrics. Dr. Cassel is past President of the American College of Physicians and past Chair of the American Board of Internal Medicine. In 1997–1998, she was a member of the President's Advisory Commission on Consumer Protection and Quality in the Health Care Industry. She chairs the boards of trustees of the American Board of Internal Medicine, The Greenwall Foundation, and the Ethics Advisory Panel for the Kaiser Permanente Health System. She is also a trustee of the Russell Sage Foundation. Dr. Cassel has served on several IOM committees, most recently as Chair of the Committee on Care at the End of Life.

William Ching is a student at the New York University School of Medicine. His research focuses on mechanisms of development of molecular specialization at the node of Ranvier during myelination in the mammalian nervous system. He is the medical student/resident physician representative to the Council on Graduate Medical Education, an advisory council of the U.S. Department of Health and Human Services. He has served in various leadership roles in organized medicine, including the executive boards of the Medical Society of the State of New York and the New York County Medical Society, as well as the House of Delegates of the American Medical Association (AMA). He has been involved in efforts to achieve universal access to health care, co-founding the Children's Health

Insurance Initiative of the AMA Medical Student Section.

Marilyn P. Chow is Vice President, Patient Care Services, California Division, for Kaiser Permanente. She is also Program Director for The Robert Wood Johnson Foundation Executive Nurse Fellows Program. Previously, Ms. Chow was Vice President, Patient Care Services, for Summit Medical Center, and Dean for Clinical Affairs, Samuel Merritt College, in Oakland, California. She was appointed by the mayor to the San Francisco City and County Social Services Commission and served as its president for 2 years. Ms. Chow is recognized for her expertise in the regulation of nursing practice, workforce policy, and primary care. She has received several awards, including the American Nurses Association's (ANA) Ethnic Minority Women's Honors in Public Health and the University of California, San Francisco, School of Nursing's Distinguished Alumni Award. Ms. Chow is currently a member of the National Advisory Council on Nurse Education and Practice, the Hartford Institute for Geriatric Nursing, the editorial advisory board of *Nurse Week*, and the California Office of Statewide Health Planning's Technical Advisory Committee. She is also a fellow of the AAN, and was recently appointed as the At-Large Nursing Representative to the Joint Commission on Accreditation of Healthcare Organizations' Board of the Commissioner.

Stephen N. Collier is Director of the Center for Health Policy and Workforce Research and Professor of Health Science at Towson University, where he served for 9 years as Dean of the College of Health Professions. Previously, he was President and John Hilton Knowles Professor of Health Policy at the Massachusetts General Hospital (MGH) Institute of Health Professions, a graduate degree–granting institution affiliated with MGH. He has also held faculty and administrative positions at the University of Alabama at Birmingham and Georgia State

University. His current work focuses on workforce policy and studies primarily in the health professions other than medicine, with an emphasis on the allied health professions and occupations that constitute approximately one-third of the health care workforce. He has served as chairman of the Commission on Health and Human Services for the Southern Regional Education Board, a 16-state educational policy organization on whose board sits the governor of each of the member states, and as chairman of the State Policy Task Force for the Pew Health Professions Commission. A fellow of the Association of Schools of Allied Health Professions (ASAHP), he has held fellowships as an Education Policy Fellow with the Institute for Educational Leadership and a Kellogg/ASAHP Health Policy Fellow. Dr. Collier has a Ph.D. in political science.

John D. Crossley is Vice President for Operations and Nursing Practice and Head, Division of Nursing, at the University of Texas M. D. Anderson Cancer Center, where he is responsible for all patient care and support service operations needed to deliver and manage care in the inpatient setting. His prior experience includes serving in nursing executive roles at University Hospitals of Cleveland, The University of Iowa Hospitals and Clinics, and Thomas Jefferson University Hospital; as emergency department nurse manager at Johns Hopkins; and as critical care staff nurse at the University of Michigan Medical Center. He has presented original research on the nurse executive role, its relation to institutional governing bodies, and implications for nurse executives. While at University Hospitals of Cleveland, Dr. Crossley was Executive Director of The Robert Wood Johnson Foundation/Pew Charitable Trust Strengthening Hospital Nursing grant. He is a member of the National Advisory Council on Nurse Education and Practice of the Health Resources and Services Administration, U.S. Department of Health and Human Services. Dr. Crossley was recently named to the Oncology Nursing Society Steering Council. He is a consultant to the University of Texas System, Center of Excellence Grant for Patient Safety, Agency for Healthcare Research and Quality.

Robert S. Galvin is Director of Global Health Care for General Electric. He is in charge of the design and performance of GE's health programs, totaling more than $2 billion annually, as well as being responsible for GE's medical services, which encompass more than 1 million visits in GE clinics in over 20 countries. Dr. Galvin has focused on issues of market-based health policy and financing, with a special interest in developing a business case for quality. He is a past member of the Strategic Framework Board and a current member of the Strategic Advisory Committee to the National Quality Forum. He is currently on the Board of the National Committee for Quality Assurance and is Vice-Chairman of the Washington Business Group on Health. He is a founding member of the Leapfrog Group, sponsored by the Business Roundtable in Washington, D.C. Dr. Galvin has published widely on issues affecting the purchaser side of health care and is an Associate Professor Adjunct of Medicine at Yale, where he directs a seminar series on the private sector for The Robert Wood Johnson Foundation Clinical Scholars fellowship. He is a fellow of the American College of Physicians.

Carl J. Getto is Senior Vice President for Medical Affairs/Associate Dean for Hospital Affairs of the University of Wisconsin Hospital and Clinics. He has previously been Dean and Provost at Southern Illinois University School of Medicine, Professor of Psychiatry and Vice Dean at the University of Wisconsin (UW) Medical School, and Associate Dean/Director of Clinical Affairs at the UW Hospital and Clinics in Madison. He currently serves as Chair of the Council on Graduate Medical Education. His administrative experience at UW included serving as Acting Dean of the Medical School, Acting Chair of the Department of Psychiatry, Director of the university's pain treatment program, and Director of the Psychiatry

Consultation Service for both UW and Middleton Veterans Administration Hospital. In November 2000, Dr. Getto was appointed to chair the Governor's Task Force on Medical Errors.

Robin Ann Harvan is Director of the Office of Education of the University of Colorado Health Sciences Center (UCHSC). She has extensive experience in the design, development, implementation, and evaluation of curricula and instructional materials, with emphases in ethics education and communication in health and medicine. Before coming to UCHSC, she was Associate Professor and Chair of the Department of Interdisciplinary Studies at the University of Medicine and Dentistry of New Jersey (UMDNJ) and Director of the Graduate Program in Health Professions Education, sponsored jointly by UMDNJ and Seton Hall University-College of Education and Human Services. Dr. Harvan has held numerous leadership positions in professional organizations related to health professions education and has contributed significantly to the field through her publications and national presentations.

Polly Johnson is Executive Director of the North Carolina Board of Nursing. She is administrator of the Nurse Licensure Compact in North Carolina and a member of the compact administrators group for those states implementing this new licensure model for multistate practice. Prior to her appointment as Executive Director, she served as Practice Consultant with the Board and as Associate Director of Practice. Ms. Johnson has held nursing administration positions in tertiary-level care, as well as in home health. Her administrative activities have included the development and implementation of practice standards, quality assurance programs, and patient classification and productivity systems, as well as personnel and fiscal management. In addition, she has experience as a clinical nurse specialist and program coordinator in an ambulatory care setting, in which she designed and implemented interdisciplinary clinical programs in several specialty areas. Ms. Johnson holds an adjunct academic appointment in the School of Nursing, University of North Carolina at Chapel Hill. She chaired the Unlicensed Assistive Personnel Task Force at the National Council of State Boards of Nursing in 1997–1998 and presently serves on other regulatory advisory panels. She also serves on several statewide task forces related to health care for the citizens of North Carolina. She is a frequent presenter at both the state and national levels on nursing regulation for the 21st century.

Robert L. Johnson (IOM) is Professor and Chair of Pediatrics, Director of Adolescent and Young Adult Medicine, and Professor of Psychiatry at the University of Medicine and Dentistry of New Jersey, New Jersey Medical School. Dr. Johnson's interest and activities focused on adolescents have resulted in his participation in a multitude of local, state, and national organizations. He has also served as a member of the boards of many organizations whose activities are directed at the adolescent. He has published widely and conducts an active schedule of teaching, research, and clinical practice at the New Jersey Medical School. Dr. Johnson has previously served as an IOM committee member for the Immunization Finance Dissemination Workshop and is a member of the Health Care Services Board.

David Leach is Executive Director, Accreditation Council for Graduate Medical Education. He is certified in internal medicine and endocrinology, and underwent additional training in pediatric endocrinology. His work is focused primarily on chaordic organizations, the teaching of improvement skills, and the aligning of accreditation with emerging health care practices. Dr. Leach is past Assistant Dean at the University of Michigan, primarily directing the Henry Ford Health System experiences for Michigan students, and Director of Medical Education at Henry Ford, playing a role in the

affiliation between that institution and Case Western Reserve University School of Medicine. While at Case Western University, Dr. Leach was instrumental in implementing an innovative curriculum for medical residents, which was recognized and supported by The Robert Wood Johnson Foundation and the Pew Charitable Trust Partnerships. He was awarded the Good Samaritan Award by Governor John Engler for his work over 25 years at a free clinic in Detroit.

Judy Goforth Parker is Professor in the Department of Nursing at East Central University. She is also a member and current co-chair of the National Advisory Council on Nursing Education and Practice (NACNEP), member of the AIDS Advisory Board of the U.S. Department of Health and Human Services, member of the Joint NACNEP and Continuing Graduate Medical Education Committee, and member of the National Tribal Diabetes Advisory Workgroup of the Indian Health Service. She is a past grant reviewer for the U.S. Department of Health and Human Services, Division of Nursing. She is a legislator for the Chickasaw Nation and has devoted much of her work to improving the quality of health care for Indians with diabetes.

Joseph E. Scherger (IOM) is Dean of the College of Medicine at Florida State University in Tallahassee. Dr. Scherger came to FSU from the University of California-Irvine College of Medicine, where he was Associate Dean for Primary Care and Professor and Chair of the Department of Family Medicine. His many years practicing medicine include serving as a migrant health physician in the National Health Service Corps, running his private practice in California, and serving as Vice President for Family Practice and Primary Care Education at Sharp HealthCare in San Diego. Dr. Scherger is a past fellow in the Kellogg National Fellowship Program, in which he focused on health care reform and quality of life. His awards include Family Physician of the Year by the American Academy of Family Physicians; Outstanding Clinical Instructor in the School of Medicine at the University of California, Davis; the Thomas W. Johnson Award for Family Practice Education; and the AAMC Humanism in Medicine Award. He is a past President of the Society of Teachers of Family Medicine and currently serves on the Board of Directors of the American Board of Family Practice and the Society of Teachers of Family Medicine. Dr. Scherger was elected to the IOM in 1992 and served as a member of the IOM committee studying Quality of Health Care in America and the subcommittee on Building the 21st Century Health System.

Joan Shaver is currently Professor and Dean, College of Nursing, at the University of Illinois at Chicago (UIC). At UIC, she serves as Co-Director for the National Center of Excellence in Women's Health Research Core. Formerly at the University of Washington School of Nursing, Dr. Shaver was Professor and Department Chair, Co-Director of the Center for Women's Health Research, and Faculty Liaison Director for an academia/ corporate partnership for older adult care though the School of Nursing. Dr. Shaver has conducted funded research in women's health for over 15 years. She and her team were among the first to study sleep problems as part of menopause transition. Dr. Shaver has an abiding interest in nursing advancement, leadership development, and the shaping of health systems. Through the UIC Nursing Institute, she and colleagues bring leaders together across various health care sectors for the annual Power of Nursing Leadership event. She has served as consultant to the University of Hong Kong, as well as to novice investigators from, and as program reviewer for, several universities. She is a fellow at the American Academy of Nursing and a member of Sigma Theta Tau International.

David Swankin is President and CEO of the Citizen Advocacy Center. He is also a partner in the law firm of Swankin and Turner. Mr. Swankin has a broad background in both government and public interest advocacy. He has provided legal services to numerous public interest and professional organizations, including the National Association of Consumer Agency Administrators, the National Consumers League, and the Consumer Federation of America. Previously, Mr. Swankin was a Deputy Assistant Secretary at the U.S. Department of Labor. He was the first Executive Director of the White House Office of Consumer Affairs. He was also a member of the original National Advisory Council to the Consumer Product Safety Commission. He served as a Commissioner on the Pew Health Professions Commission during 1997 and 1998. Mr. Swankin is the recipient of the 1999 Lillian D. Terris Award for Distinguished Board Service in enhancing public and professional understanding of the missions of credentialing organizations and the meaning associated with professional credentials.

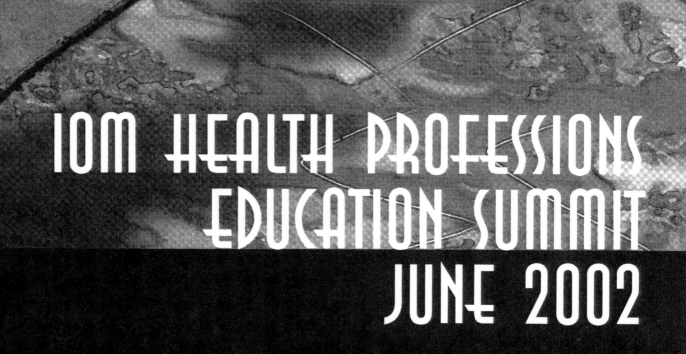

IOM HEALTH PROFESSIONS EDUCATION SUMMIT
JUNE 2002

AGENDA, STRATEGIES, AND PARTICIPANTS

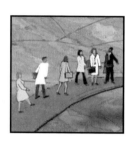

Appendix B
Health Professions Education Summit Agenda

JUNE 17, 2002

9:00 Welcome and Introductions

Edward Hundert, Organizing Committee Co-Chair, and Dean and Professor, School of Medicine and Dentistry, University of Rochester

Mary Wakefield, Organizing Committee Co-Chair, and Director, Center for Rural Health, School of Medicine & Health Sciences, University of North Dakota

Sam Shekar, Associate Administrator for Health Professions and Assistant Surgeon General, Health Resources and Services Administration (HRSA)

Carolyn Clancy, Acting Director, Agency for Healthcare Research and Quality (AHRQ)

Harry Kimball, President and CEO, ABIM Foundation

9:20 Quality Initiatives at the Institute of Medicine

Kenneth Shine, President, Institute of Medicine

Janet Corrigan, Director, Board on Health Care Services, Institute of Medicine

9:40 "Crossing the Quality Chasm" and Preparing the Health Professions Workforce

William Richardson, President and Chief Executive Officer, W. K. Kellogg Foundation

10:00 Questions and Answer session for Kenneth Shine and William Richardson

10:15 Break

10:25 **Panel Discussion**
Patient-Centered Care and the Chronically Ill: What Does the Future Hold?

Moderator: ***J. Lyle Bootman,*** Dean, College of Pharmacy, University of Arizona

Panelists: ***Robert Galvin,*** Director Global Health, General Electric; ***Mary Naylor,*** Professor in Gerontology Nursing, School of Nursing, University of Pennsylvania; ***William Stead,*** Director of the Informatics Center, Associate Vice Chancellor for Health Affairs, Vanderbilt University; ***Myrl Weinberg,*** President, National Health Council

> Advances in informatics, genetics, and other scientific areas are posed to change the nature of clinical practice. How are such advances making care more patient-centered for the chronically ill and what's on the horizon? What are the implications for health professions education?

12:05 **Questions and Answers for Panelists**

12:15 **Keynote Address: Call to the Health Professions**
Don Berwick, President and CEO, Institute for Healthcare Improvement

Question and Answers For Don Berwick

12:45 **Plenary Session Adjourns**
Working Group Sessions & Lunch

1:30 **General Session**
Overview of Group Assignments and Tasks

Edward Hundert and *Mary Wakefield*, Organizing Committee Co-Chairs

1:35 **Identifying Strategies and Devising Action Plans**

Bob King, President and CEO, Goal QPC

> Unique problem-solving methods to generate and prioritize strategies and related action plans will be presented.

1:45 **Interdisciplinary Small Working Groups**
Identifying Strategies for Reform

> Pre-assigned, facilitated working groups (based largely on participant preference) will work on generating next steps for health professions education reform with respect to the following areas: Patient-Centered Care, Evidence-Based Practice, Informatics, Interdisciplinary Teams, and Quality Improvement.

5:15 **General Session**
Review Day One and Present Plan for Day Two

Edward Hundert and *Mary Wakefield*, Organizing Committee Co-Chairs

JUNE 18, 2002

8:45 **General Session**
Review Plan for Day Two and Present Select Key Strategies From Day One

Edward Hundert and *Mary Wakefield*, Organizing Committee Co-Chairs

---

9:15 **Interdisciplinary Small Working Groups**
Create And Finalize Action Plans Around Key Strategies

> Participants will select their choice of facilitated working groups based on where they themselves can most directly contribute.

1:00 **Working Lunch**

1:45 **General Session**
Report Critical Key Actions to General Session

> Leaders of each group will present selected breakthrough action steps to general session.

2:15 **Questions and Answers for Working Group**

2:30 **Break**

2.45 **Panel Discussion**
Key Action Steps: What are the Policy and Regulatory Implications?

Moderator: **Edward Hundert,** Dean and Professor, University of Rochester School of Medicine

Panelists: **Ross Baker,** Health Administration, University of Toronto; **Bob Berenson**, Senior Consultant, AcademyHealth; **Dan Duffy**, COO, ABIM; **Charles Inlander**, President, People's Medical Society; **Joey Ridenour**, President, National Council of State Boards of Nursing; **Colleen Conway Welch**, Dean of Nursing, Vanderbilt; **Don Williams**, Executive Director, Washington Board of Pharmacy.

3:45 **QUESTION AND ANSWERS**

4:00 **General Session**
Synthesis of Major Next Steps, Action Plans, and Closing Remarks

Edward Hundert and *Mary Wakefield*, Organizing Committee Co-Chairs

---

4:15 **Adjourn**

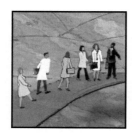

Appendix C

Summit Strategies and Actions

The following summarizes proposed strategies developed by participants at the Institute of Medicine's Health Professions Education Summit held in June 2002 to integrate the core set of competencies set forth in this report into health professions education. These strategies address distinct but overlapping groups—oversight experts, health care academic and practice leaders, health professions faculty, and researchers—and apply to all disciplines. The committee reviewed the ideas that emerged from the seven interdisciplinary groups at the summit and identified the following five cross-cutting strategies:

- Define a common language and core competencies across the professions.

- Integrate the core competencies into oversight processes (accreditation, licensing, and certification).

- Motivate and support leaders, and monitor the progress of the overall reform effort.

- Develop evidence-based curricula and teaching approaches as they relate to the core set of competencies.

- Develop faculty as teaching/learning experts in the core set of competencies.

The committee carefully considered the ideas generated by the 150 expert participants at the summit in developing this follow-up report and its recommendations.

Box C-1. Method for Generating Potential Strategies and Actions

Proposed strategies and related actions were developed at a 2-day summit by 150 experts who worked in small groups through a facilitated process known as Hoshin. Hoshin (Kanri), developed in Japan, is a collection of tools and techniques used in strategic planning, which builds on the U.S. techniques of management by objectives and quality improvement (see Chapter 1). Committee members provided guidance to the 20 professional facilitators who coached summit participants in generating proposed strategies, actions, and implementation tactics using this process.

The Hoshin method was selected for the summit because it relies on a proven approach used by leaders in health care—the plan, do, study, and act cycle; requires active and equal participation by all involved; and enables the identification of "breakthrough" strategies that the participants believe will make it possible to leverage the best results and should thus be carried out first (Counsell et al., 1999; Hyde and Vermillion, 1996; Platt and Laird, 1995).

The following sections present an overarching vision developed by the committee for each of these proposed strategies and a specific articulation of the strategy by individuals in the respective summit group. Actions are also presented, most at the national level, that represent ways the strategies could be implemented by one or more participants in each group. Finally, select institutional-level actions, developed by individuals from the listed organizations are included for illustrative purposes.

DEVELOP A COMMON LANGUAGE AND CORE COMPETENCIES

Vision

Across health professions schools and practice environments, there is a shared definition of key terms and competencies for educating health care professionals. While the roles of individual health professionals vary with respect to each of the competencies, these shared definitions transcend occupations and enable cross-disciplinary communication. They enable interdisciplinary groups to define and reach consensus around a core set of competencies for health professions education.

Proposed Strategy and Actions Identified by Individuals in the Common Language and Competencies Working Group

Proposed Strategy

The health professions should collectively take deliberate steps to build consensus around common terms and competencies.

Proposed Actions

- Initiate a formal process, involving a broad cross section of disciplines, to identify areas of agreement and those that are sensitive or taboo. Also, identify how terms are used in the literature, oversight processes, law, and policy. Write a paper identifying related issues.

- Engage key stakeholder professions in understanding the problems and related issues associated with the lack of a common language.

- Create an interdisciplinary group to develop a common language.

- Define commonalities with respect to competencies across professions, and capture in a report.

The common language and common competency working group included representation from:

- Alliance for Continuing Medical Education

- American Nurses Association, Division of Nursing

- Case Western Reserve University, School of Nursing

- Colorado Chapter of the Federation of Families for Children's Mental Health

- East Central University

- Grace Episcopal Church

- Health Resources and Services Administration, Office of Rural Health Policy

- Intermountain Health Care Inc., Clinical Support Services

- The Johns Hopkins University Hospital, Nurse Administration, GYN/OB

- Mayo Clinic, Department of Nursing

- National Network of Health Career Programs in Two-Year Colleges

- University of Missouri-Columbia, School of Health Professions

- University of Texas, M.D. Anderson Cancer Center, Nursing Practice and Policy

- Yale University, Managed Behavioral Health Care, Department of Psychiatry

Selected Institutional Actions

- Contact National Board for Certification in Occupational Therapy (NBCOT) to brief them on summit objectives and discuss possible future role

- University of Texas, M.D. Anderson Cancer Center contact office of nursing services for nominees for group focused on developing common language and survey Texas Medical Center leadership for how to link this effort to professional partnership project.

- Alliance for Continuing Medical Education, Colorado Chapter of the Federation of Families for Children's Mental Health, National Network of Health Career Programs in Two Year Colleges, create a list of individuals to participate on the interdisciplinary team charged with developing common competencies.

INTEGRATE CORE COMPETENCIES INTO OVERSIGHT PROCESSES

Vision

There is consistency in approach and coordination across the various health professions oversight organizations—including accrediting, licensing and certification bodies—as the result of a focus on an agreed-upon set of core competencies. This consistency allows for enhanced communication, integration, and synergy within and across oversight bodies and professions. As a result, educational programs are evaluated based on outcomes, and a clinician's competency is assessed upon entry into practice and regularly throughout his or her career.

Proposed Strategy and Actions Identified by Individuals in the Integrating Competencies into Oversight Processes Working Group

Proposed Strategy

The IOM should convene accreditation, licensing, and credentialing organizations across the spectrum of health professions to move all health professions to competency-based oversight that incorporates the five core competencies.

Proposed Actions

- Establish communication links among regulators.
- Define accreditation standards and measurements for the core competencies. Share best practices across professions.
- Request the addition of the competencies to licensing exams.
- Develop model oversight processes related to the competencies.

The oversight process working group included representatives from:

- AcademyHealth
- Accreditation Council for Continuing Medical Education
- Accreditation Council for Graduate Medical Education
- Alliance of Community Health Plans

- American Association of Colleges of Nursing
- American Board of Internal Medicine
- American College of Clinical Pharmacy
- American Council on Pharmaceutical Education
- American Osteopathic Association
- Association of American Medical Colleges, Educational Standards
- Baton Rouge General Medical Center, Family Medicine Residency Program
- Baystate Medical Center
- Center for Clinical Improvement, Vanderbilt University
- Charles R. Drew University of Medicine-Los Angeles, Dean's Office/ Academic Affairs
- Citizen Advocacy Center
- Commission on Accreditation of Allied Health Education
- Federation of State Medical Boards of the United States, Inc.
- The George Washington University, Department of Health Policy
- Harvard School of Public Health

- Holy Cross Hospital, Continuing Medical Education
- Joint Commission on Accreditation of Healthcare Organizations
- National Association of Boards of Pharmacy, Washington State Board of Pharmacy
- National Board of Medical Examiners
- National Council of State Boards of Nursing
- National Institute for Standards in Pharmacist Credentialing
- National Organization for Associate Degree Nursing
- National Organization of Nurse Practitioner Faculties
- North Carolina Board of Nursing
- People's Medical Society
- School of Nursing, Vanderbilt University
- The Robert Wood Johnson Foundation, Communications Department
- Donald W. Reynolds Department of Geriatrics, University of Arkansas Medical Sciences
- University of Washington, MEDEX

Selected Institutional Actions

- Develop National Council of State Boards of Nursing model regulations for quality improvement competencies.
- Work on developing and defining standards for quality improvement for practicing pediatricians as part of maintenance of certification at the American Board of Pediatrics.
- Request the addition of informatics competencies to the pharmacy licensing exam by the National Association of Boards of Pharmacy.
- Joint Commission on Accreditation of Healthcare Organizations advocate and participate in a meeting of regulators across the health professions.
- Federation of State Medical Boards work with the National Board of Medical Examiners to incorporate patient-centered care skills into the United States Medical Licensing Exam.

Motivate And Support Leaders And Monitor Progress Of Reform Effort

Vision

An interdisciplinary group of education leaders—from practice environments and academic and continuing education settings, and including students—works to create a shared mission and vision for health professions education that relates to but is larger than the five competencies. This reform-minded group monitors progress made on integrating the competencies into health professions education and provides a regular status report to the larger education and quality communities. The group also supports leadership training for education leaders, recognizes and rewards leaders who make a significant contribution to educational reform, and continuously assesses changing skill needs for health professionals.

Proposed Strategies and Actions Identified by Individuals in the Leadership and Monitoring Working Groups

Proposed Strategies

The IOM should convene a council of national educational leaders in academic and practice settings, as well as leading consumer advocacy organizations, to develop a joint agenda related to leadership and the overarching vision of a prepared health professional, and to monitor progress against this vision.

The health professions should collectively identify funds that can be used to foster and support partnerships between education and practice leaders with regard to the overarching vision of a prepared health professional.

Proposed Actions

- Develop and make use of fact sheets and case studies that make the case for the overarching vision and the need for reform of health professions education.

- Promote the overarching vision to the leadership of key organizations.

- Monitor, evaluate, and communicate progress against this vision by examining efforts to integrate the core competencies into health professions education, including the extent to which summit participants fulfill their commitments.

- Make the case to sponsors for funding of the council, leadership development activities, and partnerships between academic and practice leaders.

- Create and support leadership development skills programs, including efforts to link academic and practice leaders.

- Create and fund fellowships for formal leadership courses.

- Charge the IOM to create a national award related to implementation of the overarching vision.

The leadership and monitoring progress working group included representation from:

- American Nurses Association

- American Board of Internal Medicine Foundation

- American Organization of Nurse Executives

- American Pharmaceutical Association

- American Psychological Association

- Association of Academic Health Centers

- Association of Schools of Allied Health Professions

- Center for Innovation in Public Mental Health, University of South Carolina

- College of Nursing, University of Iowa

- Continuing Medical Education, Greensboro Area Health Education Center

- Department of Family and Preventive Medicine, University of Utah School of Medicine

- Department of Nursing and Patient Services, Shands Hospital at the University of Florida

- Department of Veterans Affairs, Veterans Health Administration

- Drugay and Associates

- General Electric Co.

- Grantmakers in Health

- Healthcare Education Industry Partnership, Minnesota State Colleges and Universities

- John A. Hartford Foundation

- The Johns Hopkins University

- Kaiser Permanente

- Kansas University School of Nursing

- Massachusetts General Hospital

- National Association of Community Health Centers

- National Association of Hispanic Nurses

- National Center for Healthcare Leadership

- The Robert Wood Johnson Foundation, Executive Nurse Fellows Program

- National Committee for Quality Assurance

- School of Nursing, Duke University

- School of Nursing, Oregon Health Sciences University

- School of Nursing, University of Michigan

- St. Cloud State University

- University of Rochester, School of Medicine and Dentistry

- University of Wisconsin Hospital and Clinics, University of Wisconsin Medical School

- Vanderbilt Medical Center

- Virginia Commonwealth University

- Wake Area Health Education Center, University of North Carolina Chapter

Selected Institutional Actions

- National Association of Community Health Centers provide leadership development related to integrating the summit vision of health professions education into community health center boards.

- National Center for Healthcare Leadership revise graduate and continuing education curricula to be consistent with the vision in the *Quality Chasm* report (Institute of Medicine, 2001).

- Implement new skills in experiential learning and in continuing education for pharmacists at the Area Health Education Center in Wake, North Carolina.

- Minnesota Healthcare Education Industry Partnership convene a working group on implementation of the overarching summit vision.

- Create a coalition of all five University of Iowa health science deans, chief executive officers of hospitals and hygienic laboratories, and provosts to develop state-level legislative strategies to support the summit's overarching vision.

Develop Evidence-Based Curricula And Teaching Approaches

Vision

A rich, readily available evidence base exists to make the case for teaching the five competencies to health professions students and clinicians, demonstrating the strong relationship between these competencies and enhanced quality outcomes for patients. This evidence base is integrated across all the health professions through linkages to profession-specific databases. In addition, those who instruct and mentor health professionals—in both academic and continuing education settings—have access to a well-developed evidence base regarding the effectiveness of teaching methods and a continuously updated best-practices database.

Proposed Strategies and Actions Identified by Individuals in the Developing Evidence-based Curricula and Teaching Approaches Working Groups

Proposed Strategies

Educate health professional groups to focus on the link between health professions education and quality.

Activate health professional groups to create and fund a new organization whose research efforts are focused on evidence-based education and the five competencies.

Proposed Actions

- Promote the link between education and quality within leading health professional organizations.

- Key medical organizations focus on this link as an important issue; begin by writing an editorial to make the case.

- Association of Academic Health Centers or National Academies of Practice bring health educational professionals together to address the redesign of education, specifically organizational structures.

- Ask the National Quality Forum to examine the relationship between education and quality.

- Strengthen the focus of fellowships on the overarching vision defined by the IOM committee.

- Investigate/identify information systems that support evidence-based education.

- Establish an Interdisciplinary Health Professional Education organization, supported by key stakeholders, to identify and evaluate education models that further the overarching vision, function as a repository of related data, and disseminate best practices. This organization should:

  - Demonstrate the importance of education by focusing on compelling examples in which educational interventions have made a difference to patient outcomes (e.g., wrong-side surgeries, diabetes).

  - Perform a systematic review of the literature (e.g., best evidence in medical education or best-evidence medical practice, and determine a future research agenda, looking to the Agency for Healthcare Research and Quality.

  - Conduct a best-practice review of universities that have integrated the five competencies into their curricula to understand what they do and how/why it is a best practice.

  - Create a database of best practices in health professions education.

  - Develop research collaboratives among institutions to demonstrate the effectiveness of the five competencies in both academic and continuing education settings.

  - Assess the interest among the leadership of the American Academy of Family Physicians in hosting a symposium as part of the research agenda–setting process.

**The evidence base and curricula development
working groups included representation from:**

- ABIM Foundation
- AcademyHealth
- American College of Healthcare Executives
- American College of Physicians
- American Hospital Association
- American Society of Internal Medicine
- Cedars Sinai Medical Center
- Community College of Philadelphia, Department of Nursing
- Council on Graduate Education
- Creighton University, Office of Interprofessional Education
- Florida State University, College of Medicine

- Health Resources and Services Administration, Division of Medicine and Dentistry, Bureau of Health Professions
- New Jersey Medical School, University of Medicine and Dentistry of New Jersey, Division of Adolescent and Young Adult Medicine
- North American Association of Medical Education and Communication Companies
- Nurse Practitioner Faculty
- Oregon Health and Science University, School of Medicine
- The Robert Graham Center: Policy Studies in Family Practice and Primary Care

- University of Arizona, Arizona Health Sciences Center, College of Pharmacy

- University of Iowa, College of Nursing

- University of Maryland, Department of Medical and Research Technology, School of Medicine

- University of Massachusetts, School of Nursing

- University of Missouri, School of Medicine

- Veterans Health Administration, Department of Veterans Affairs

- Veterans Health Administration, National Center for Patient Safety

Selected Institutional Actions

- For the American College of Physicians, American Society of Internal Medicine, project on Training for Quality and Evidence Base, stimulate and write educational articles for publication in Annals of Internal Medicine.

- North American Association of Medical Education and Communication Companies (NAMMEC), with support from the NAAMEC Board, develop a research project proposal focused on creating a model for evaluating the effectiveness of continuing medical education, carry out the project, and then disseminate results at meetings and in publications.

- Robert Graham Center: Policy Studies in Family Practice and Primary Care approach the Agency for Healthcare Research and Quality, the National Science Foundation, Health Resources and Services Administration, and foundations about sponsoring a symposium to develop a research focus on interdisciplinary education.

- Creighton University, Office of Interprofessional Education, design and conduct an interdisciplinary collaborative research project on effective evaluation of interprofessional education.

- Texas Tech University Health Sciences Center, School of Nursing, identify specific content for an interdisciplinary curriculum through a survey of faculty in various professions at Texas Tech.

- Center for Health Policy and Workforce Research, Towson University, hold a follow-up meeting with Towson University leadership to identify resources and plan the development of new centers and cross-professional activities.

- University of Alabama at Birmingham (UAB), School of Health Related Professions, create a center or office for health professions education and workforce development at UAB.

- Samford University, McWhorter School of Pharmacy, distribute a "Samford Plan" (continuous quality improvement process model for curriculum development and refinement) to all summit participants.

Develop Faculty As Teaching And Learning Experts

Vision

Faculty development programs exist at the national and regional levels for the array of health professional educators, focused on the overarching vision presented in this report. The programs, many of which are interdisciplinary, prepare faculty to convey the five competencies, as well as to adopt an evidence-based approach to education.

Proposed Strategy and Actions Identified by Individuals in the Developing Faculty As Teaching and Learning Experts Working Group

Proposed Strategy

Health professional groups should motivate and enable faculty in their efforts to implement the overarching vision of a prepared health professional.

Proposed Actions

- Identify cross-cutting faculty competencies.

- Help organize an inventory of best practices and resources for faculty development.

- Create a program to recognize "educational scholars" on a national basis, and promote the program to health professional schools.

- Develop and disseminate online self-instructional lessons/courses in faculty development related to the overarching vision.

- Help develop models for reform of criteria for promotion and related compensation, including tenure models, starting initially in the field of pharmacy.

The faculty development working group included representation from:

- American Association of Colleges of Pharmacy

- Community College of Philadelphia, Department of Nursing

- Health Resources and Services Administration

- Michigan State University

- National League for Nursing

- New York University, School of Medicine

- Southern Regional Education Board, Council on Collegiate Education for Nursing

- University of Colorado Health Sciences Center, Office of Education

- University of Washington, School of Medicine

- Virginia Commonwealth University, School of Nursing

Selected Institutional Actions

- School of Medicine, New York University, assess existing quality improvement processes for education as part of an effort to achieve consensus on a quality improvement model for all of health professions education.

- Council on Collegiate Education for Nursing, Southern Regional Education Board (SREB), conduct a validation study of expected competencies for nurse educators in 16 SREB states.

- American Association of Colleges of Pharmacy help organize an effort to inventory best practices and resources for faculty development.

- Virginia Commonwealth University provide information technology orientation for new faculty.

- Michigan State University work with a national professional training organization and the Association of Program Directors in Internal Medicine to begin to develop online self-instruction in faculty development.

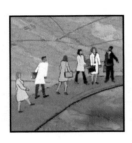

Appendix D
Attendee List

Virginia Adams
School of Nursing
University of North Carolina at Wilmington

Eula Aiken
Council on Collegiate Education for Nursing
Southern Regional Education Board

Eleni Anagnostiadis
National Insitute for Standards in Pharmacist
Credentialing

Kathleen Andreoli
College of Nursing
Rush-Presbyterian-St. Luke's Medical Center

Ross Baker
Department of Health Policy, Management and
    Evaluation
University of Toronto

Ruth Ballweg
MEDEX
University of Washington

Stan Bastacky
Health Resources and Services Administration

Jim Battles
Center for Quality Improvement and Patient Safety
Agency for Healthcare Research and Quality

Carol Bazell
Division of Medicine and Dentistry
Health Resources and Services Administration

Geraldine Bednash
American Association of Colleges of Nursing

Cynthia Belar
American Psychological Association

Bruce Bellande
Alliance for Continuing Medical Education

Jim Bentley
American Hospital Association

Bob Berenson
AcademyHealth

Sharon Bernier
Nursing
Montgomery College at N-OADN

Donald Berwick
Institute for Healthcare Improvement

Claudia Beverly
Donald W. Reynolds Department of Geriatrics
University of Arkansas of Medical Sciences

Brian Biles
Department of Health Policy
The George Washington University

Marian Bishop
Department of Family and Preventive Medicine
University of Utah School of Medicine

Maxine Bleich
Ventures in Education, Inc.

Mark Boesen
Public Affairs
The American Health Quality Association

Linda Bolton
Cedars Sinai Medical Center

J. Lyle Bootman
College of Pharmacy
Arizona Health Sciences Center
University of Arizona

Eileen Breslin
School of Nursing
University of Massachusetts

Kathleen Buckwalter
College of Nursing
University of Iowa

Roger Bulger
Association of Academic Health Centers

Helen Burstin
Center for Primary Care Research
Agency for Healthcare Research and Quality

Carol Bush
Clinical Support Services
Intermountain Health Care, Inc.

Forrest Calico
Office of Rural Health Policy
Health Resources and Services Administration

Patricia Calico
Health Resources and Services Administration

Theresa Carroll
School of Nursing
University of Texas Health Science Center at Houston

Christine Cassel
School of Medicine
Oregon Health and Science University

James Cawley
The George Washington University

William Ching
School of Medicine
New York University

Peter Chodoff
Jefferson Medical Center

Marilyn Chow
Kaiser Permanente

Nancy Clark
College of Medicine
Florida State Unviersity

Peter Coggan
Henry Ford Hospital

Jordan Cohen
Office of the President
Association of American Medical Colleges

Elaine Cohen
Bureau of Health Professions
Health Resources and Services Administration

Stephen Collier
Center for Health Policy and Workforce Research
Towson University

Colleen Conway-Welch
School of Nursing
Vanderbilt University

John Coombs
School of Medicine
University of Washington

John Crossley
Division of Nursing
M. D. Anderson Cancer Center
University of Texas

Byron Crouse
American Academy of Family Physician

Thomas Curtin
National Association of Community Health Centers

Joseph Dean
McWhorter School of Pharmacy
Samford University

James Delk
Vanderbilt Medical Center

Don Detmer
Cambridge University

Charlotte Dey
Grace Episcopal Church

Richard Diamond
Center for Biologics Evaluation and Research
U.S. Food and Drug Administration

Marge Drugay
Drugay and Associates

Dan Duffy
ABIM

Jack Ebeler
Alliance of Community Health Plans

Ronald Edelstein
Dean's Office/Academic Affairs
Drew University of Medicine and Science

Noel Eldridge
National Center for Patient Safety
Veterans Health Administration

Tom Elwood
Association of Schools of Allied Health Professions

Ives Erickson
Massachusetts General Hospital

Chris Esperat
School of Nursing
Health Sciences Center/Texas Tech University

Bill Finerfrock
National Association of Rural Health Clinics

Sondra Flemming
Commission on Accreditation of Allied Health
    Education

Mary Fralic
The Johns Hopkins University

Paul Friedmann
Baystate Medical Center

Doreen Frusti
Department of Nursing
Mayo Clinic

Robert Galvin
General Electric Co.
Yale University School of Medicine

Carole Gassert
Department of Nursing
Bureau of Health Professions
Health Resources and Services Administration

Denise Geolot
Department of Nursing
Bureau of Health Professions
Health Resources and Services Administration

Carl Getto
University of Wisconsin Medical School
University of Wisconsin Hospital and Clinics

John Gosbee
National Center for Patient Safety
Veterans Administration

Murray Grant
Continuing Medical Education
Holy Cross Hospital

Marjorie Grimsley
Colorado Chapter of the Federation of Families for
    Children's Mental Health

Jerry Grossman
Lion Gate Management Corporation

Atul Grover
Graduate Medical Education Branch
Division of Medicine and Dentistry
Health Resources and Services Administration

Debra Gussman
Jersey Shore Medical Center

Karen Hackett
American College of Healthcare Executives

Kristofer Hagglund
School of Health Professions
University of Missouri-Columbia

Deborah Hales
Department of Education
American Psychiatric Association

Denise Harmening
Department of Medical and Research Technology
    School of Medicine
University of Maryland

Robin Harvan
Office of Education
University of Colorado Health Sciences Center

Linda Headrick
School of Medicine
University of Missouri

Tim Henderson
Institute for Primary Care and Workforce Analysis
National Conference of State Legislatures

Madeline R. Hess
Nursing Special Initiatives and Program Systems
    Branch
Health Resources and Services Administration

Michael Hoge
Managed Behavioral Health Care, Department of
    Psychiatry
Yale University

Denise Holmes
Association of Academic Health Centers

Edward Hundert
Case Western Reserve University

Charles Inlander
People's Medical Society

George Isham
Health Partners

Bonnie Jennings
American Academy of Nursing/American Nurses
    Foundation
Institute of Medicine Nurse Scholar in Residence

Polly Johnson
North Carolina Board of Nursing

Robert Johnson
Division of Adolescent and Young Adult Medicine
New Jersey Medical School at University of Medicine
    and Dentistry of New Jersey

Harold Jones
School of Health Related Professions
University of Alabama at Birmingham

Judy Miller Jones
National Health Policy Forum
The George Washington University

Kristin Juliar
Healthcare Education Industry Partnership
Minnesota State Colleges and Universities

Harry Kimball
ABIM Foundation

Ken Kizer
National Quality Forum

Murray Kopelow
Accreditation Council for Continuing Medical
    Education

William Lang
American Association of Colleges of Pharmacy

Daniel Laskin
School of Dentistry
Virginia Commonwealth University

David Leach
Accreditation Council for Graduate Medical
    Education

Lucian Leape
Harvard School of Public Health

Larry Lewin
Executive Consultant

Judith Lewis
School of Nursing
Virginia Commonwealth University

Elizabeth Mahaffey
National Organization for Associate Degree Nursing

Lucinda Maine
American Association of Colleges of Pharmacy

Paul Mazmanian
Virginia Commonwealth University

Andrea Mengel
Department of Nursing
Community College of Philadelphia

Cheryl Merritt
Occupational Therapist

Laurinda Merritt
Family Medicine Residency Program
Baton Rouge General Medical Center

Paul Miles
Center for Clinical Improvement
Vanderbilt University

Jolene Miller
National Network of Health Career Programs in
    Two-Year Colleges

Karen Miller
Kansas University School of Nursing

Pamela Mitchell
Biobehavioral Nursing and Health Systems
University of Washington

Lucy Montalvo-Hicks
Council on Graduate Medical Education

Shirley Moore
School of Nursing
Case Western Reserve University

John Morris
Center for Innovation in Public Mental Health
University of South Carolina

Jennifer Muldoon
AcademyHealth

Mary Naylor
School of Nursing
University of Pennsylvania

Elizabeth Nelson
American College of Physicians
American Society of Internal Medicine

Brenda Nevidjon
School of Nursing
Duke University

Don Nielsen
American Hospital Association

Linda Norman
School of Nursing
Vanderbilt University

Richard O'Brien
Office of Interprofessional Education
Creighton University

Peggy O'Kane
National Committee for Quality Assurance

Angella Olden
Nurse Administration, GYN/OB
The Johns Hopkins University Hospital

Marian Osterweis
Association of Academic Health Centers

Ann O'Sullivan
National Organization of Nurse Practitioner Faculties

Thomas O'Toole
Community Campus Partnerships for Health
The Johns Hopkins University

Judy GoForth Parker
East Central University

Greg Pawlson
National Committee for Quality Assurance

Nilda Peragallo
National Association of Hispanic Nurses

Cheryl Peterson
American Nurses Association

Robert Phillips
The Robert Graham Center: Policy Studies in Family
    Practice and Primary Care

Sally Phillips
Bureau of Health Professions
Agency for Healthcare Research and Quality

Stephanie Pincus
Department of Veterans Affairs
Veterans Health Administration

Walter Pories
North Carolina State Medical Board
East Carolina University

John Porter
Hogan & Hartson, L.L.P.

Kathleen Potempa
School of Nursing
Oregon Health Sciences University

Jane Radford
Continuing Medical Education
Geensboro AHEC

William Richardson
W. K. Kellogg Foundation

Cathy Rick
Department of Veterans Affairs
Veterans Health Administration

Joey Ridenour
National Council of State Boards of Nursing

Elena Rios
National Hispanic Medical Association

Rose Rivers
Department of Nursing and Patient Services
Shands Hospital at the University of Florida

Laura Robbins
John A. Hartford Foundation

Joseph Scherger
College of Medicine
Florida State University

Anne Schwartz
Grantmakers in Health

Paul Schyve
Joint Commission on Accreditation of Healthcare
    Organizations

Peter Scoles
National Board of Medical Examiners

Joan Shaver
College of Nursing
University of Illinois at Chicago

Vickie Sheets
National Council of State Boards of Nursing

Marie Sinioris
National Center for Healthcare Leadership

Carl Sirio
Critical Care Medicine
University of Pittsburgh

Yvonne Small
School of Nursing
University of Michigan

Harrison Spencer
Association of Schools of Public Health

William Stead
Vanderbilt University

David Stevens
Educational Standards
Association of American Medical Colleges

Linda Stierle
American Nurses Association

John Studach
National Center for Health Fitness

David Sundwall
American Clinical Laboratory Association

David Swankin
Citizen Advocacy Center

Paul Tarini
Communications Department
The Robert Wood Johnson Foundation

Humphrey Taylor
The Harris Poll

George Thomas
American Osteopathic Association

James Thompson
Federation of State Medical Boards of the United
    States, Inc.

Pamela Thompson
American Organization of Nurse Executives

Richard Tischler
North American Association of Medical Education
    and Communication Companies

Toyin Tofade
Wake AHEC
University of North Carolina Chapter

Theresa "Terry" Valiga
National League for Nursing

Peter Vlasses
American Council on Pharmaceutical Education

Mary Wakefield
Center for Rural Health
School of Medicine and Health Sciences
University of North Dakota

Susan Warner
St. Cloud State University

Edwin Webb
American College of Clinical Pharmacy

Myrl Weinberg
National Health Council

Mike Whitcomb
Association of American Medical Colleges

Donald Williams
Washington State Board of Pharmacy
National Association of Boards of Pharmacy

Susan Winckler
American Pharmaceutical Association

Daniel Wolfson
ABIM Foundation

Douglas Wood
American Association of Colleges of Osteopathic
    Medicine

Michael Zaroukian
Michigan State University